IMPROVE YOUR SLEEP IN 14 DAYS

Words Charlotte Haigh
Additional writing Hannah Ebelthite, Trish Leslie
Images iStock

Editor Mary Comber
Art Director Lucy Pinto
Chief Sub-editor Eve Boggenpoel

Publisher Steven O'Hara
Publishing Director Dan Savage
Marketing Manager Charlotte Park
Commercial Director Nigel Hole

Printed by Acorn Web Offset Ltd, Normanton, West Yorkshire

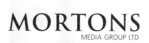

Published by Mortons Media Group Ltd,
Media Centre, Morton Way,
Horncastle, LN9 6JR
01507 529529

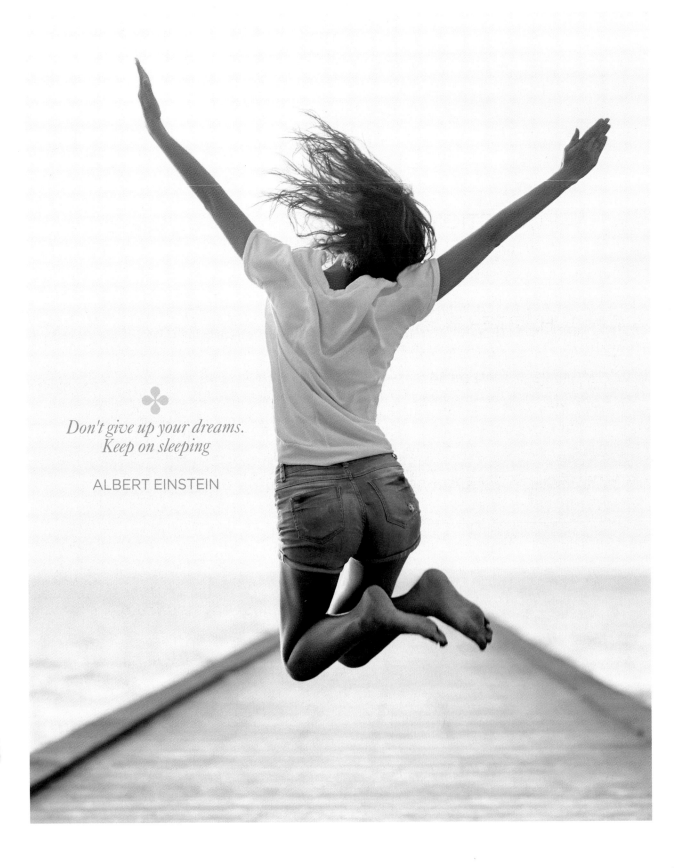

Don't give up your dreams.
Keep on sleeping

ALBERT EINSTEIN

Contents

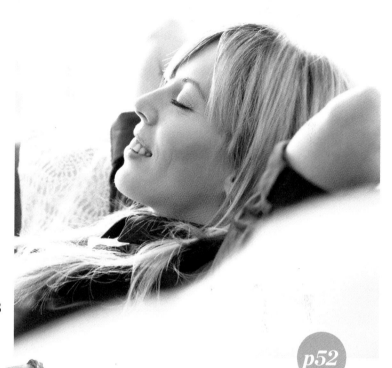

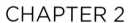

p52

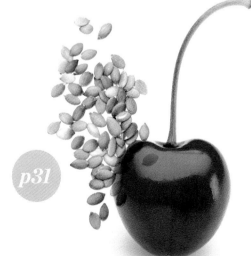

p31

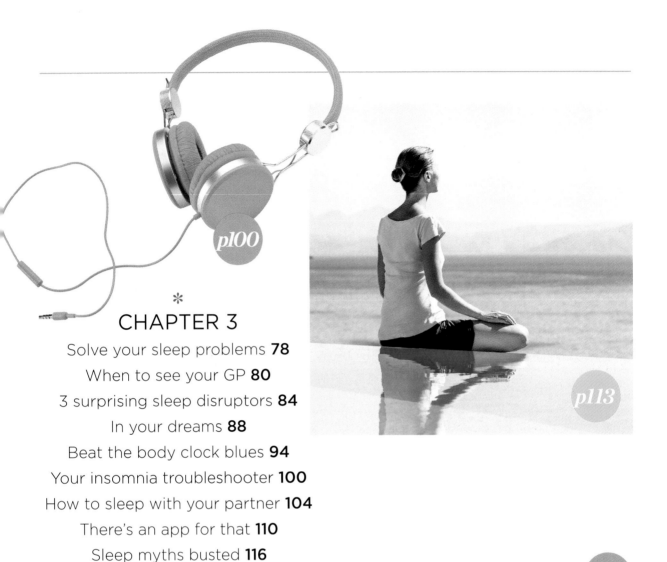

p100

p113

p76

*

CHAPTER 3

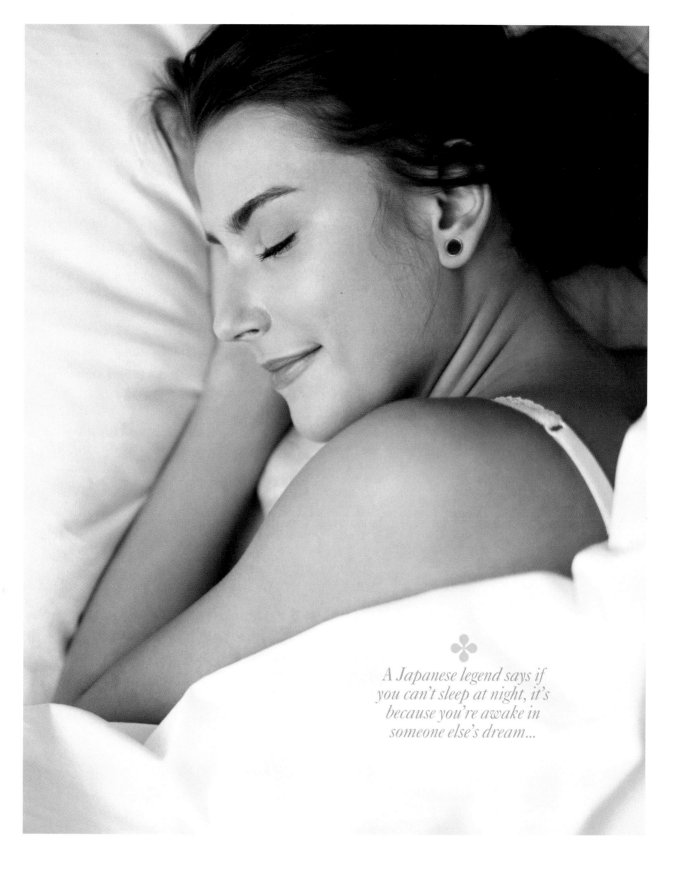

A Japanese legend says if you can't sleep at night, it's because you're awake in someone else's dream...

Welcome

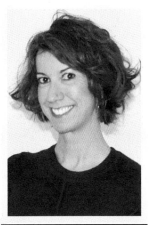

We all know the power of a great night's sleep – how positive, calm and refreshed it leaves you feeling. Your eyes sparkle, your skin glows and your whole day seems to flow better. Unfortunately, for many of us, a perfect night's sleep is elusive. The irony, of course, is that when life's tough, sleep is essential for helping you cope. Even if you don't have full-blown insomnia, you may be plagued by what's known as 'junk sleep' – where you don't have enough, or it's poor quality, so you never wake feeling refreshed. And a stressful situation is magnified by tiredness – find out exactly why sleep matters so much on p14.

As a health journalist, I'm lucky to have access to leading sleep experts, tips and techniques for quality shuteye. Over the years, I've made it a bit of a mission to gather the best information and try to put it into practice – and the good news is there are strategies that really work! From creating the perfect snooze-inducing atmosphere in your bedroom (p32) to beating those bad habits that keep you awake (p42), some of the simplest tricks can really make a difference. Having a great night's sleep isn't just about what you do before you go to bed, either – your whole day can have an impact on your slumber. Find out how on p68. And if it's your pesky mind that's keeping you awake with overthinking, discover how to soothe stress-related sleep problems on p54. Those nights you find yourself staring at the ceiling? Turn to our insomnia troubleshooting guide on p100.

I hope you find the advice and tricks in this book transform your sleep. Keep going – it can take a while to change habits and reap the benefits. Here's to banishing those dark circles for good!

Charlotte Haigh
Author of *Improve Your Sleep in 14 days*

THE AUTHOR

Charlotte Haigh is a freelance health journalist who contributes to a wide range of national newspapers and magazines, as well as writing for charity websites and communications agencies. She has a special interest in psychology and emotional wellbeing. In her spare time, Charlotte enjoys fiction-writing and yoga.

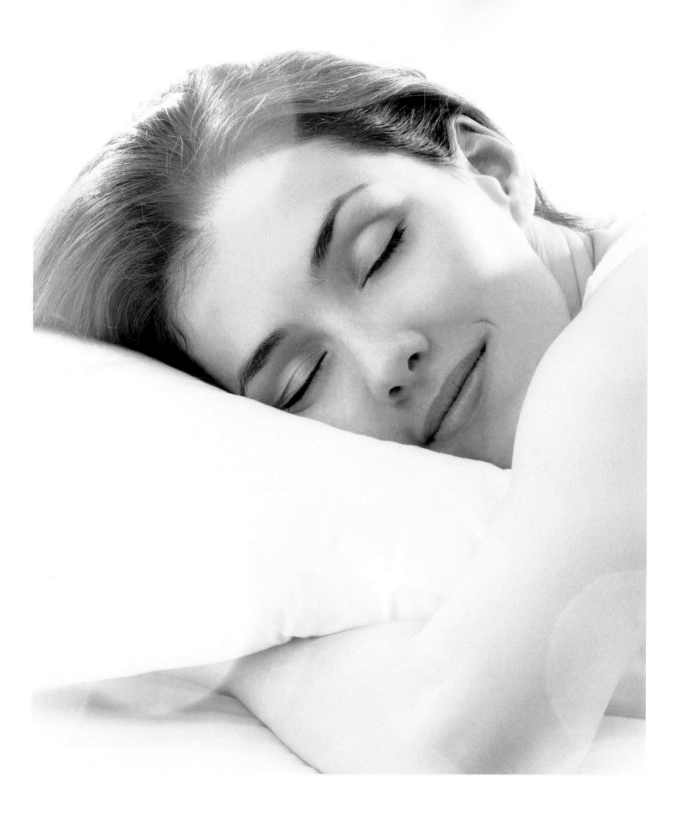

How to use this book

Looking forward to a good night's rest? Read these instructions to make sure you get all the benefits of your 14-day plan!

Do you struggle to fall asleep, lie awake in the night with a racing mind or always wake up feeling tired? You're not alone. More and more people are suffering from insomnia and disrupted sleep. But the good news is, with a few simple lifestyle changes you can enjoy an unbroken night's rest – every night! We've compiled all the latest, science-backed advice into an easy 14-day plan that's guaranteed to help improve your slumber. Here's how to get started.

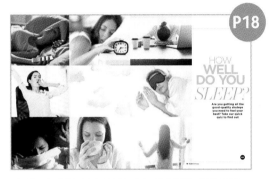

1. DISCOVER YOUR SLEEP STYLE

What sort of sleeper are you? Take our quiz to help understand your sleep pattern and pinpoint the areas you need to focus on to get a better night's rest.

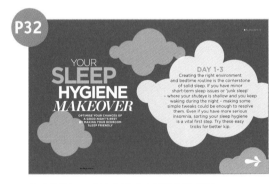

2. TRY A SLEEP MAKEOVER

Having the right sleep environment and bedtime routine is the foundation to sound slumber. Learn how to beat your bad sleep habits, create a relaxing sanctuary and discover 10 surprising sleep fixes you can put in place straight away.

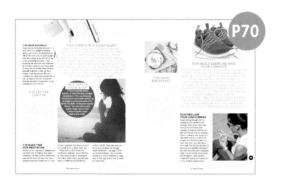

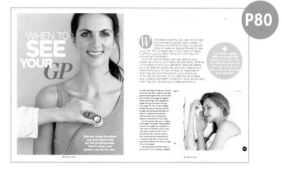

3. CHANGE YOUR LIFESTYLE

Getting a good night's sleep isn't just about what you do at bedtime. Follow our timetable for the perfect sleep-friendly day. Try some snooze-inducing yoga poses to help calm your system and discover the natural remedies that help you drift off.

4. SOLVE YOUR SLEEP PROBLEMS

Once you've put a sleep-friendly lifestyle in place, it's time to tackle those stubborn sleep thieves. Find out if you could benefit from medical support, and discover other useful helpers – from sleep retreats to handy apps – that can come to your rescue.

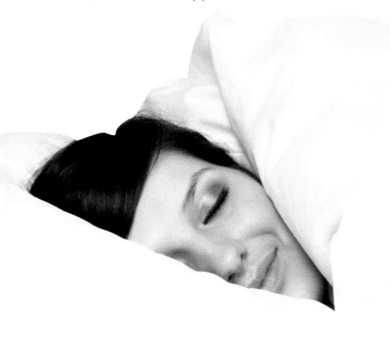

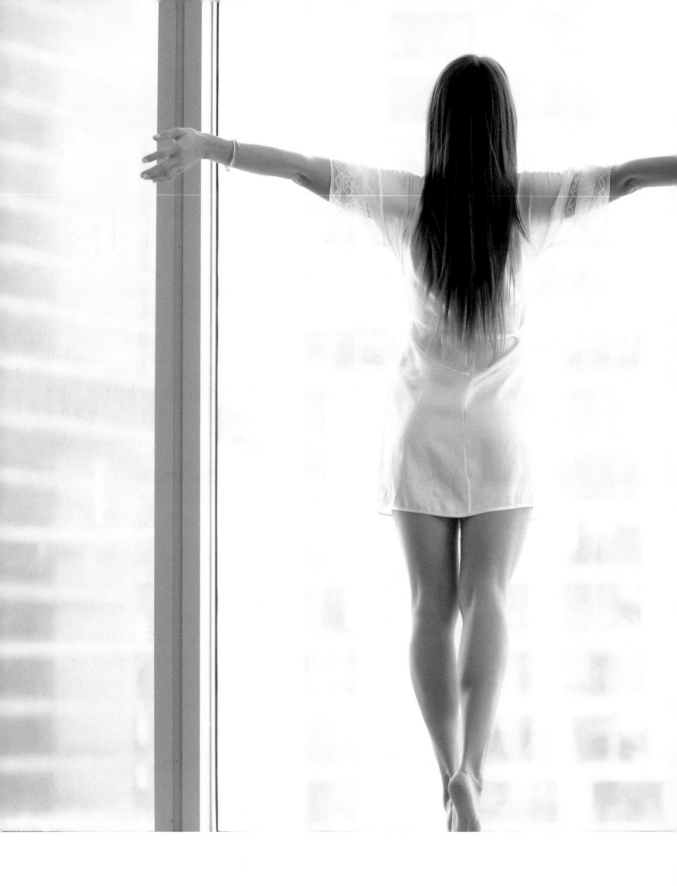

DISCOVER YOUR
SLEEP STYLE

Yes, we're all different. Your friend may be able to sleep like a log on a plane after downing three espressos, while you may struggle to nod off in the comfort of your own bed, even after sipping chamomile tea since 5pm. The following pages will help you work out exactly how to sleep well – including the tweaks to make to your bedroom and routine (p32) and the bad habits to break (p42). And if you never wake feeling refreshed, our quiz (p18) will help you establish whether you're getting less sleep than you realise. Understanding your sleep pattern and making a few simple steps to start improving it is the first step to perfect shuteye.

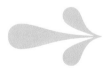

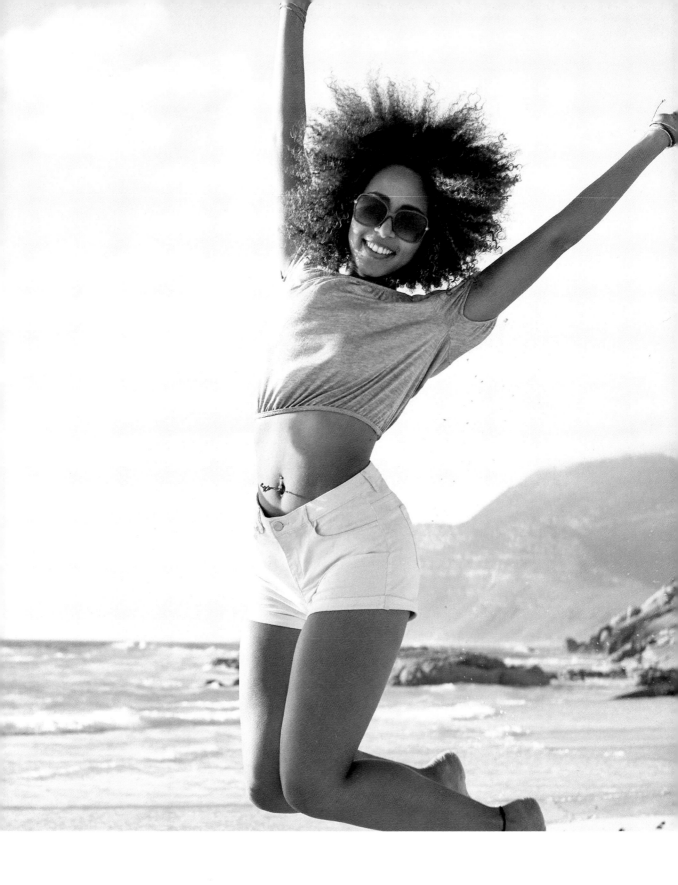

WHY
SLEEP
MATTERS

Not just vital for giving you enough energy – sleep is crucial for your health and wellbeing too

Most of us don't get enough sleep. Research by the Mental Health Foundation shows one-third of us experience insomnia – and according to the Economic and Social Research Council, one-in-10 of us now regularly take medication to help us sleep. But lack of sleep doesn't just cause a frayed temper and red eyes – it also affects your health. Here's why solid shuteye really counts.

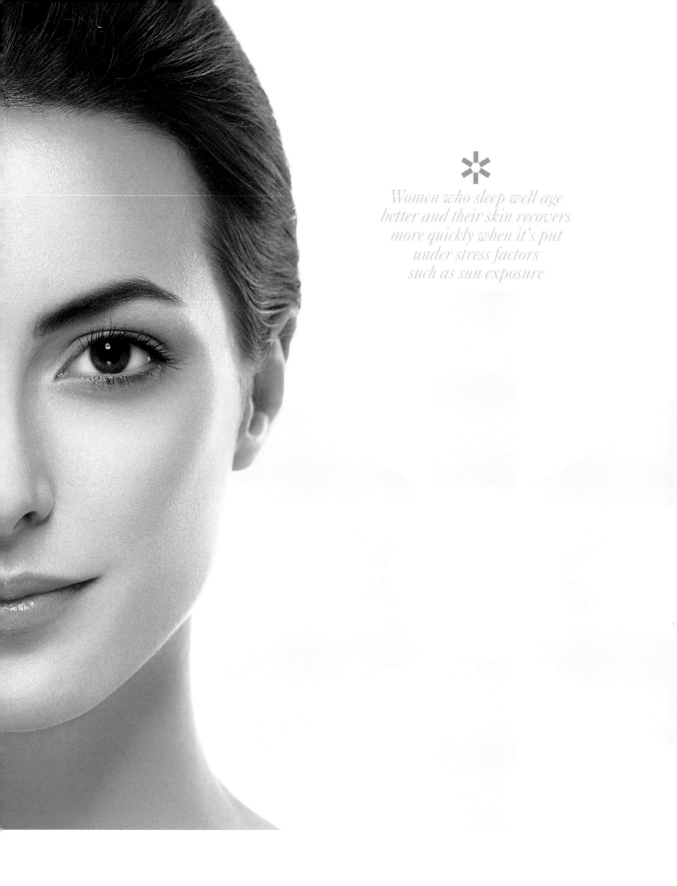

Women who sleep well age better and their skin recovers more quickly when it's put under stress factors such as sun exposure

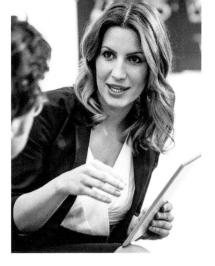

1. IT REALLY IS BEAUTY SLEEP

You've probably noticed your skin looks fresher and brighter when you go to bed early. A study from University Hospitals Case Medical Center in Cleveland, Ohio, US, found women who sleep well age better, and their skin recovers more quickly when it's put under stress factors such as sun exposure. Plus, poor sleepers have more signs of skin ageing, including wrinkles, sagging and pigmentation.

2. IT KEEPS YOUR MIND SHARP

Getting good-quality sleep can help lower your risk of dementia, according to US research. The scientists think that during sleep, your brain gets 'cleaned' – and substances called beta-amyloid plaques, linked with Alzheimer's, are cleared away. Miss out on sleep and there's an increased risk of plaques building up.

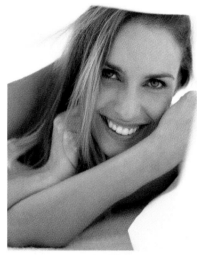

3. IT MAY REDUCE CANCER RISK

Some research is showing a link between poor sleep and some common forms of cancer. One study found sleeping for less than six hours a night puts you at a 50 per cent increased risk of bowel cancer. And other research has linked lack of sleep with more aggressive breast cancer. Doctors believe poor kip disturbs your immune system and can trigger dangerous inflammation inside your body. And it may be that the hormone melatonin, produced when you sleep, could help prevent cell damage that can lead to cancer.

4. IT BOOSTS YOUR IMMUNE SYSTEM

Studies on shift workers reveal a great deal about how lack of sleep damages your immune system. Daylight, which triggers wakefulness, is a stronger influence than even a deep need for sleep, so most shift workers average only five to five-and-a-half hours of sleep. Constantly over-riding your bodyclock's signals creates a lot of stress in your body, which can dampen immunity. A study from the American Academy of Sleep Medicine found sleeplessness causes a spike in white blood cells in a bid to boost immunity, which is the same way your body reacts to high stress. A recent study found sleep helps to strengthen your immune system's memory – so it's better able to remember bugs it's come across before, and mount a more effective defence against them.

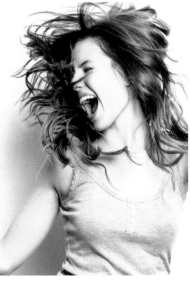

5. IT KEEPS YOU SLIM

People who sleep badly are more likely to be overweight. A study from the University of Stanford, in the US, found poor sleep leads to raised levels of ghrelin, a hormone that makes you feel hungry, and lower levels of leptin, another hormone linked with feelings of satiety. That's why you may have found you eat more after a bad night's sleep. Get enough and you'll have much more control over what you eat.

6. IT CUTS YOUR RISK OF HEART DISEASE

If you regularly wake up feeling unrested due to poor sleep, you're at 63 per cent higher risk of cardiovascular disease, according to research. A study by the American Heart Association found that sleeping for fewer than six hours a night increases inflammatory substances in the blood by 25 per cent, raises blood pressure and heart rate, and affects blood sugar levels, which can raise your risk of heart disease and type 2 diabetes. Sufficient sleep will lower your risk.

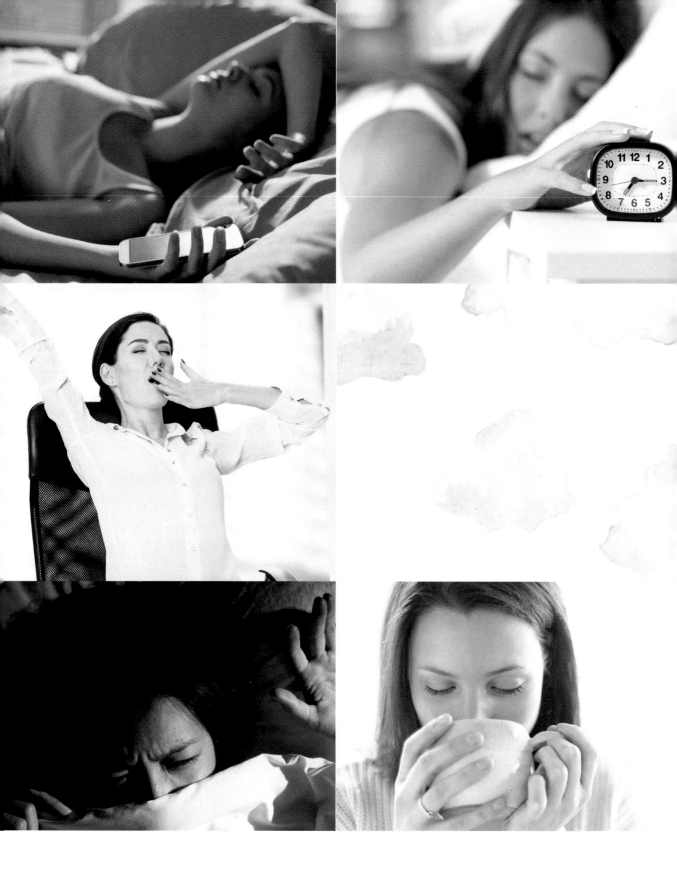

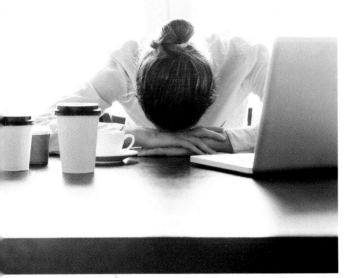

HOW
WELL
DO YOU
SLEEP?

Are you getting all the good-quality shuteye you need to feel your best? Take our quick quiz to find out

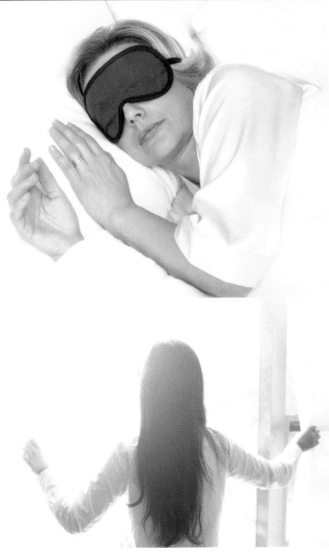

1. HOW MANY HOURS' SLEEP WOULD YOU SAY YOU GET A NIGHT, ON AVERAGE?

Ⓐ Eight hours or more
Ⓑ Five to eight hours usually
Ⓒ Rarely more than five, sometimes zero

2. DO YOU THINK YOU GET THE SLEEP YOU NEED TO FUNCTION AT YOUR BEST THE NEXT DAY?

Ⓐ Yes, I don't think I need more
Ⓑ I think I could do with a bit more or better quality sleep
Ⓒ Definitely not

3. HOW DO YOU FEEL EMOTIONALLY WHEN YOU'VE HAD A BAD NIGHT'S SLEEP?

Ⓐ Tired but not too worried – I'll make up for it the next night
Ⓑ I feel grouchy and exhausted all day and take some extra steps to get to bed early
Ⓒ I feel wired and anxious, and worry I'll get stuck in a pattern of sleeping badly

4. DO YOU GO TO BED AS SOON AS YOU FEEL TIRED IN THE EVENINGS?

Ⓐ Yes, I start getting ready for bed when I feel sleepy
Ⓑ I try to but there are often jobs (or a TV programme) to finish off first
Ⓒ I'm always tired

5. DO YOU HAVE TROUBLE FALLING ASLEEP AT NIGHT?

Ⓐ No, I read for a bit, turn out the light and nod off
Ⓑ Sometimes, if I'm worried about something
Ⓒ Most nights, yes

6. YOU HAVE A LOT GOING ON. HOW DOES IT AFFECT YOUR SLEEP?

Ⓐ Not too much – I can usually sleep whatever's happening in my life
Ⓑ I have some bad nights but that's partly because I don't prioritise sleep enough
Ⓒ My sleep is the first thing to go when I'm stressed or excited

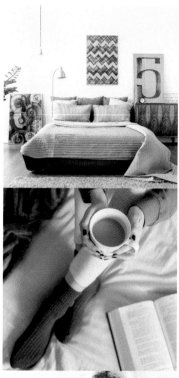

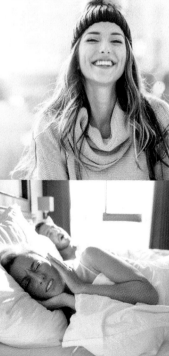

7. DO YOU WAKE AT NIGHT AND FIND IT HARD TO SLEEP AGAIN?

Ⓐ No, I generally sleep through undisturbed
Ⓑ Occasionally
Ⓒ Very often

8. DO YOU USE ANYTHING TO HELP YOU SLEEP?

Ⓐ Nothing more than a milky drink or soothing music
Ⓑ I sometimes have a nightcap or take an herbal sleep aid
Ⓒ I use prescription or recreational drugs

9. IF YOU ARE AWAKE AT NIGHT, WHAT DO YOU DO?

Ⓐ Get up, make a chamomile tea and read for a bit
Ⓑ Stay in bed, tossing and turning
Ⓒ Lie in bed feeling anxious, or scrolling through my phone

10. WHAT'S YOUR RELATIONSHIP WITH ALCOHOL?

Ⓐ I don't drink often, if at all, and then only in moderation
Ⓑ I sometimes drink to excess on a night out
Ⓒ I drink most nights, to get to sleep

10. HOW WOULD YOU RATE THE QUALITY OF YOUR SLEEP?

Ⓐ I sleep deeply and wake refreshed
Ⓑ Not bad, but not always great
Ⓒ Very poor, I sleep fitfully if at all

11. HOW WOULD YOU DESCRIBE YOUR BEDROOM?

Ⓐ My sanctuary – dark, cosy and peaceful
Ⓑ It could do with a tidy up
Ⓒ A place I associate with stress and anxiety

12. HOW WOULD YOU DESCRIBE YOUR BED?

Ⓐ Like sleeping on clouds – so comfortable
Ⓑ I wouldn't mind an upgrade
Ⓒ Old, lumpy, squeaky, too soft...

13. IF YOU'RE NOT WORKING, WHAT TIME DO YOU GET UP?

Ⓐ I naturally seem to wake around 7am
Ⓑ 9 or 10am
Ⓒ I'd just like to get to sleep in the first place

14. WHAT'S YOUR REACTION WHEN YOUR ALARM GOES OFF?

Ⓐ I turn it off and get up
Ⓑ I hit snooze once or twice
Ⓒ Panic – how am I going to get through the day on no sleep?

15. AT THE WEEKENDS, DO YOU LIE IN?

Ⓐ No, I'm up at the normal time
Ⓑ Yes, I like to get an extra hour or two if I can
Ⓒ If I eventually get to sleep, I'll lie in all morning

16. HOW DO YOU FEEL WHEN YOU GET OUT OF BED IN THE MORNING?

(A) Refreshed and ready to face the day
(B) I'm not really a morning person but I'm fine by the time I leave the house
(C) Groggy, moody and exhausted

17. AND HOW DO YOU LOOK IN THE MIRROR?

(A) Like me. Bright-eyed and rested
(B) A bit weary, but nothing a bit of concealer and blusher won't fix
(C) Birds' nest hair, dark circles and eye bags – I look how I feel

18. WHAT GETS YOU THROUGH THE MORNINGS?

(A) The yoga sun salutations and meditation I do on waking
(B) A mid-morning cuppa or two
(C) Several pots of coffee, pastries and muffins

19. DO YOU EVER FEEL SLEEPY DURING THE DAYTIME?

(A) Only if I'm jet lagged
(B) Sometimes, but I power on through with caffeine
(C) Sleepy is my default state

20. DO YOU EVER TAKE NAPS DURING THE DAY?

(A) I don't really need them, but I might power nap before a big event
(B) Does nodding off in boring meetings count?
(C) I try not to because I'm even less likely to sleep that night

21. WHAT'S YOUR EVENING WIND-DOWN ROUTINE?

(A) A light, early supper; maybe watch some TV; have a bath, then read in bed
(B) I try to turn off my phone and laptop by 10pm but don't always succeed
(C) What's a wind-down routine?

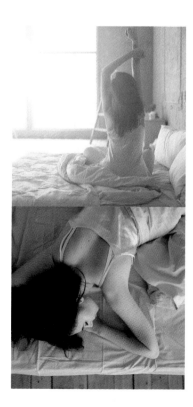

HOW DID YOU ANSWER?

IF YOU CHOSE
MOSTLY
As

IF YOU CHOSE
MOSTLY
Bs

IF YOU CHOSE
MOSTLY
Cs

Lucky you! You sleep like a baby (except babies probably wake up more). You seem to be blessed with good-quality, refreshing sleep and not to have many worries that need addressing. It could be because you have a sensible wind-down routine, consistent sleep and waking times, and you understand the value of good sleep hygiene.

There may be times in life, however, when sleep becomes more elusive. Major life changes such as having children, working evening or night shifts, sleeping with a new partner or even moving house can disrupt your routine. Periods of stress can also interfere with the quality of your slumber. You'll find lots of advice over the following pages that will help you to minimise the effects of any such changes. Learn how to calm your mind (p54), and, as someone who knows the importance of good sleep, you'll love all the expert tips, tricks, products and ideas we've compiled to help enhance your time between the sheets even more. Check out our nifty sleep apps (p110) and essential oil blends to use (p60) for a relaxing night's slumber.

You're no stranger to decent sleep – but let's face it, you're not always the best of bed fellows, either. Hopefully, answering these questions has alerted you to some of the areas where you could be more attentive to your sleep needs. It could certainly be worth keeping a diary, so you can start to identify factors that may be contributing to your some-time sleeplessness. Maybe your bedroom deserves a makeover (see p32), or perhaps your diet and lifestyle could be tweaked to help ease that morning grogginess? Check out 10 surprising sleep fixes, on p38. There's a wealth of information in this book that can help you to find the right solutions for you, and get a great night's sleep, every night.

Insomnia is clearly a very big issue for you. Perhaps you struggle to drift off, maybe you're wakeful in the night or daytime sleepiness is becoming a problem – or all three are conspiring to keep you on the brink. It would be well worth a trip to your GP to discuss your sleep difficulties (see p80). It may be that you have a sleep disorder or underlying health condition that could be resolved. Doctors don't just prescribe medication, they may be able to make referrals to other medical professionals, such as cognitive behavioural therapists, who can help you. As well as seeking outside help, you can use this book to tailor your approach to dealing with insomnia. Learn how to remove the obstacles to sleep (p84) and look back at the questions where you chose a C as your answer. These give clues as to your key areas to address if you want to improve your sleep. If you spend your weekends in bed till noon, bringing a more structured timetable in (p68) could work wonders. Each point might seem minor when you're in sleep deprivation, but the marginal gains all add up.

NIGHT OWL
OR
LARK?

It's not just a myth. People who like to stay up late or rise early have different brain structures...

Do you loathe early starts? Or do you leap out of bed in the morning without so much as a peep out of an alarm clock? Maybe you're more likely to hit the snooze button and pull the bedclothes up with a groan after staying up half the night watching a box set? Or perhaps 'early to bed, early to rise', is something that comes totally naturally to you...

It turns out that most of us really are either a night owl or an early bird. Scientists recently discovered that the physical structures of the brains of 'morning people' are different to those of us more inclined to stay up into the wee small hours. Researchers in Germany scanned the brains of those who like to stay up late, as well as early risers, and discovered that the owls' white matter was less efficient in the transmission of nerve signals than those who preferred early mornings.

BRAIN LAG

This diminished 'integrity' of the white matter, which was found in several areas of the brain, may be linked to depression, which studies have found is more prevalent among night owls. What causes it isn't yet clear, but researchers are exploring the possibility that it could be because the owls suffer from a kind of jet lag brought on by a sleep deficit. Other research has shown that owls are more likely to suffer seasonal affective disorder, although scientists don't know if there's a direct link. On the plus side, night owls can often stay focused as the day goes on.

Still, experts believe that whether you're an owl or a lark isn't set in stone. Owl or lark, more of us are tending to stay up later and later as a consequence of modern technologies and lifestyles anyway. That's largely because our biological clocks (or circadian rhythms) evolved when we had to live within the natural light-dark cycle. Modern life – and artificial light in particular – is conspiring to make us all a bit more owl-like, keeping us awake long after the sun goes down.

Research shows that the light we see in the evening can affect our biological clock, pushing us to stay awake longer. But while more of us are heading towards owl status, there are steps we can take to reset our body clocks to lark (see box right).

OWL OR LARK?

Extreme owls are often unable to sleep until 2 or 3am and true larks are up at 4 or 5am, although it's believed only about 5 per cent of us are at each extreme. According to international researchers, the bodyclock of a reasonably strong owl will be about four hours behind the equivalent lark.

BECOMING A LARK

You may not be a 'morning person' naturally, but with a little lifestyle tweaking you can change the sleeping habits of a lifetime...

✚ Get up at the same time every day. Even at weekends. And no matter how tired you feel, don't hit the snooze button.

✚ Invest in a natural daylight alarm clock. A more gentle and natural awakening than a bleeping alarm will help to reset your circadian rhythms.

✚ Exercise in the morning. Working out will boost your energy earlier in the day and could help you feel more tired sooner at night.

✚ Practise good sleep hygiene. Tap into the sleep tips on page 32 to help you nod off a little earlier – and get a restful night's sleep so you feel more refreshed in the morning.

Our biological clocks (or circadian rhythms) evolved when we had to live within the natural light-dark cycle. Modern life is conspiring to make us all a bit more owl-like

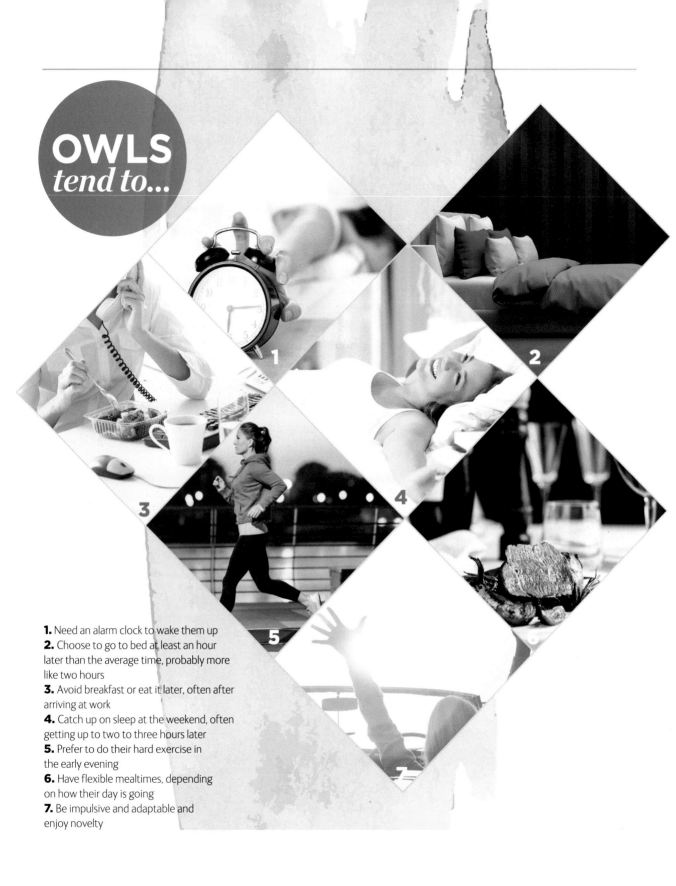

OWLS
tend to...

1. Need an alarm clock to wake them up

2. Choose to go to bed at least an hour later than the average time, probably more like two hours

3. Avoid breakfast or eat it later, often after arriving at work

4. Catch up on sleep at the weekend, often getting up to two to three hours later

5. Prefer to do their hard exercise in the early evening

6. Have flexible mealtimes, depending on how their day is going

7. Be impulsive and adaptable and enjoy novelty

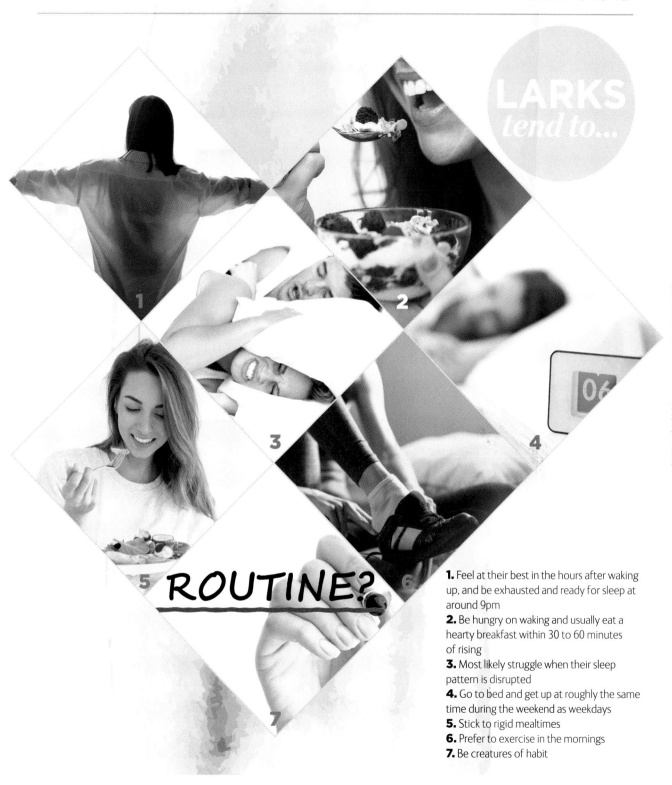

LARKS
tend to...

ROUTINE?

1. Feel at their best in the hours after waking up, and be exhausted and ready for sleep at around 9pm

2. Be hungry on waking and usually eat a hearty breakfast within 30 to 60 minutes of rising

3. Most likely struggle when their sleep pattern is disrupted

4. Go to bed and get up at roughly the same time during the weekend as weekdays

5. Stick to rigid mealtimes

6. Prefer to exercise in the mornings

7. Be creatures of habit

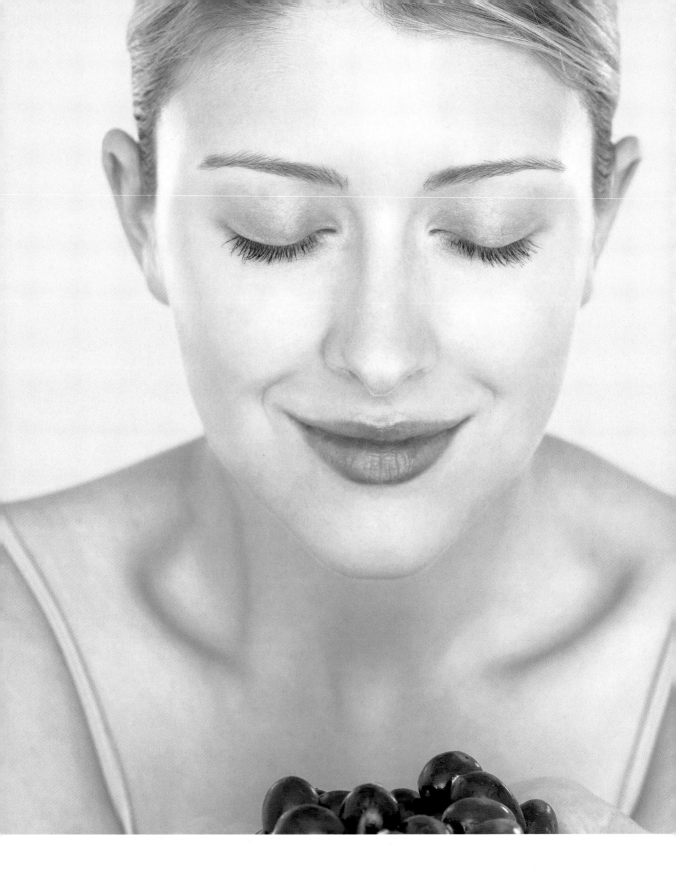

5
FOODS
TO HELP YOU
NOD OFF

**Tuck into these sleep-inducing
foods to feel sleepy fast...**

Did you know you can help ensure a good night's sleep by eating the right foods before bedtime? Some foods naturally contain chemicals and nutrients that have a soporific effect. We asked nutritional therapist Shona Wilkinson what you can eat to ensure you get a sound night's slumber.

1 TURKEY

'Turkey is often said to be a sleep-promoter, as it contains good levels of tryptophan, the amino acid that converts into serotonin and then melatonin in your body,' says Wilkinson. But it's not all about the tryptophan. Turkey is also a good source of zinc and vitamin B6 – and these, says Wilkinson, can help your body make melatonin from tryptophan. Ideally, you should have a serving of turkey earlier in the day rather than in the evening. Why not have a wholemeal pitta filled with turkey and salad for a quick lunch?

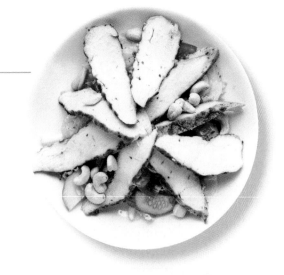

2 COCONUT WATER

Swap your hot choc for a cup of pure coconut water in the evening to help you have a restorative night's sleep. 'Coconut water is an excellent source of "electrolyte" minerals: potassium, calcium, magnesium, phosphorous and sodium,' says Wilkinson. 'Balanced levels of these minerals are needed to maintain normal muscle action, nerve function and hydration in your body. Deficiencies or imbalances may cause cramping and restless legs at night and, therefore, disturbed sleep.' Chose a natural version with no added sugars so you don't get a jolt of glucose that may disturb your kip.

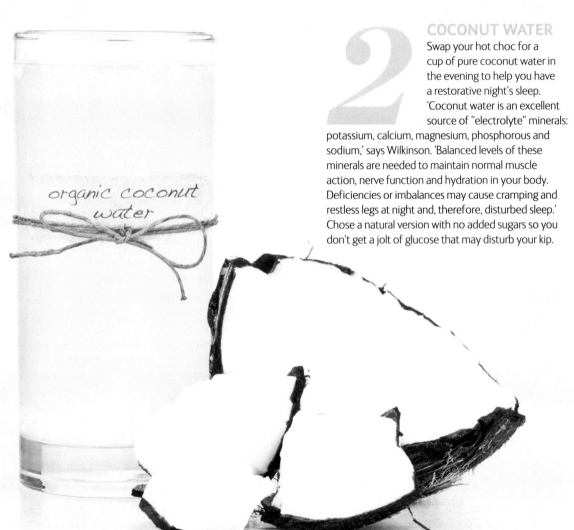

organic coconut water

3 OATS

While you're asleep, your brain and body are still using energy and need glucose to keep working. If levels fall too low, it can trigger the release of hormones adrenaline and cortisol, which can wake you up. You might also wake feeling hungry and find it hard to get back to sleep. To prevent this happening, make sure you have some slow-release carbs in the evening. 'Slow-releasing carbohydrates such as wholegrains help keep the levels of sugar (glucose) in your blood stable, providing your body with sustained energy,' says Wilkinson.

'Oats are ideal – try a small bowl of porridge or muesli, or have some oatcakes spread with nut butter as an evening snack, ideally around two hours before you go to bed. Other wholegrains have similar effects, so if you're not in the mood for oats you could try a serving of brown rice with your dinner or have a slice of rye bread spread with nut butter a couple of hours before hitting the sack. It's important to note that sugary foods and refined 'white' carbohydrates can have the opposite effect, as they quickly enter and leave the bloodstream, leaving your blood low in glucose again. So steer clear of sugary foods and white bread.'

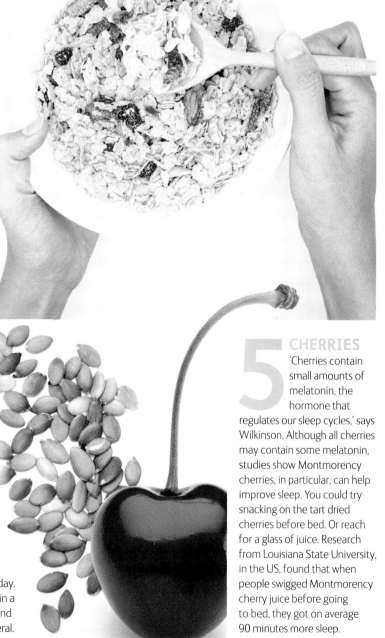

4 PUMPKIN SEEDS

'Pumpkin seeds are high in magnesium,' says Wilkinson. The mineral allows the muscle fibres in your body to relax. It's thought it also has a role in the function of the pineal gland, which produces melatonin – a hormone that regulates the sleep-wake cycle and helps you fall asleep.' Try including one to two tablespoons of magnesium-rich pumpkin seeds a day. Add to plain yoghurt, sprinkle onto salads or grind in a coffee grinder and add to porridge. All raw seeds and nuts, plus leafy green veg, are also high in the mineral.

5 CHERRIES

'Cherries contain small amounts of melatonin, the hormone that regulates our sleep cycles,' says Wilkinson. Although all cherries may contain some melatonin, studies show Montmorency cherries, in particular, can help improve sleep. You could try snacking on the tart dried cherries before bed. Or reach for a glass of juice. Research from Louisiana State University, in the US, found that when people swigged Montmorency cherry juice before going to bed, they got on average 90 minutes more sleep.

YOUR
SLEEP
HYGIENE
MAKEOVER

**OPTIMISE YOUR CHANCES OF
A GOOD NIGHT'S REST
BY MAKING YOUR BEDROOM
SLEEP FRIENDLY**

DAY 1-3

Creating the right environment and bedtime routine is the cornerstone of solid sleep. If you have minor short-term sleep issues or 'junk sleep' – where your shuteye is shallow and you keep waking during the night – making some simple tweaks could be enough to resolve them. Even if you have more serious insomnia, sorting your sleep hygiene is a vital first step. Try these easy tricks for better kip.

ENJOY THE SILENCE

Some people are used to falling asleep to the sounds of trains, planes or traffic – and, indeed, regular sounds can be comforting. That's why some people find gentle music or even white-noise recordings helpful. But for the majority of us, noise is a distraction and makes for a fitful night. Try to make your room as soundproofed as possible (think shutting the door, heavier curtains and even triple glazing). And give earplugs a go – they're especially handy if you're travelling or sharing with a snorer or noisy flatmate.

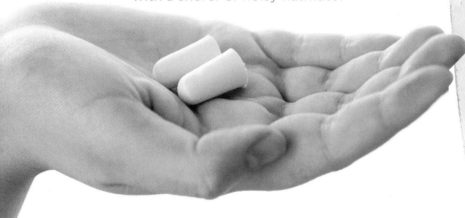

COOL IT

Studies have shown 16-17°C is the ideal temperature for sleep. 'Your body temperature cools slightly when you go to sleep, and artificially triggering this cooling can help you fall asleep,' says neuroscientist Penelope Lewis, author of *The Secret World of Sleep* (Macmillan Science, £17.99). The best way to do that? Programme your heating to switch off about an hour before bed, so your room reaches the optimal temperature by the time you hit the sack. This is also the idea behind having a warm bath before bed – it tricks your body into heating up and then cooling down again. Check how warm your duvet is – make sure you switch from a winter-weight tog to a cooler one in the summer. Make sure you don't wear too many warm clothes in bed – natural, breathable fabrics like cotton and silk are best.

SORT YOUR MATTRESS

It's well known we spend a third of our lives in bed, but when was the last time you replaced yours? If you toss and turn all night, that could be the cause. According to the Sleep Council, 68 per cent of us are sleeping in a bed that's five or more years old. Buy the biggest you can afford and consider technologies such as memory foam, which support your body well. For good advice, visit the National Bed Federation (bedfed.org.uk)

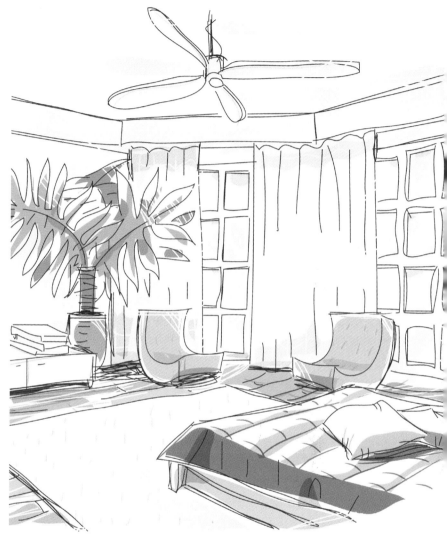

KEEP IT DARK

How light is your bedroom? 'We are hard-wired to sleep at the onset of darkness,' says clinical hypnotherapist Glenn Harrold, author of Sleep Well Every Night *(Orion, £9.99). 'Only when it's dark does your pineal gland release melatonin. Even LED light from an alarm clock or chinks of light under the door are too bright.' Invest in a blackout blind or curtains, get an analogue alarm clock that doesn't shine in the darkness and remove TVs and other light-emitting technology. A comfortable eye mask is a good option. We like the* Mulberry Silk Eye Mask, *£12.99, slumberslumber.com*

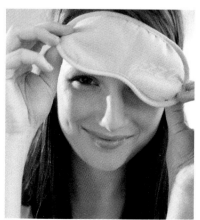

MAKE YOUR BEDROOM BEAUTIFUL

As well as keeping it cool, dark and quiet, you should make sure your bedroom is an environment that gives you pleasure. 'One of the biggest influences on how you sleep is how you actually feel about your bed and bedroom,' says Lewis. Review how you feel when you walk into it – it should be calming and comfortable. If it's messy or too brightly lit, it could be time to make some changes. And think about the décor. Soft pastel colours are considered the most soothing – lilacs, pale peaches and creams, for example. Avoid strong, bright pigments that might over-stimulate. And make sure you love the way your bed feels. Go for the best quality bed linen you can afford and make sure it's clean and crisp so you feel good getting under the duvet. Finally, don't use your bedroom for anything other than sex, sleep and gentle activities such as listening to music and gentle reading. Don't watch TV or use your laptop or mobile in bed – and keep arguments and big discussions to other rooms of your home.

TAKE TIME TO WIND DOWN

The other important aspect of sleep hygiene is taking time to relax before bed. 'Lots of us expect to fall into bed at the end of a busy day and go to sleep straight away,' says sleep researcher Dr Neil Stanley, 'but you need to give yourself time to unwind first.' Take 30-40 minutes to relax before bed. Do whatever works for you. Try a bath with some gorgeous essential oils (flick to page 60 for some soothing blends), listen to a meditation podcast, read a book (but avoid anything that stimulates your mind too much), have a warm milky drink and browse through a magazine. There aren't any rules – just do whatever helps you to feel most relaxed.

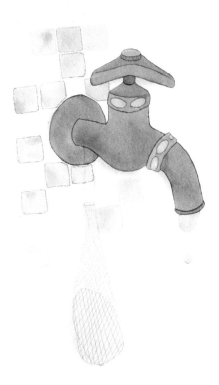

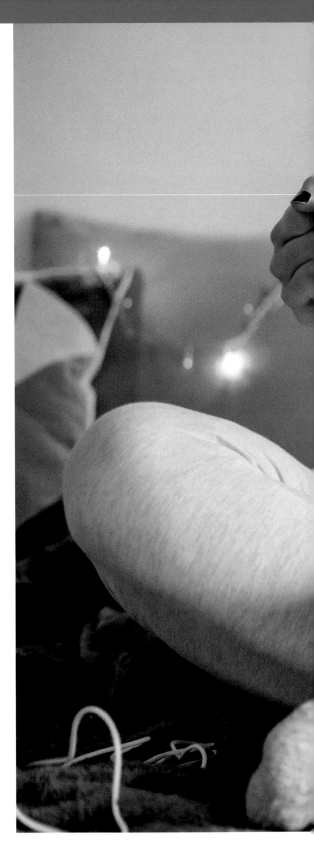

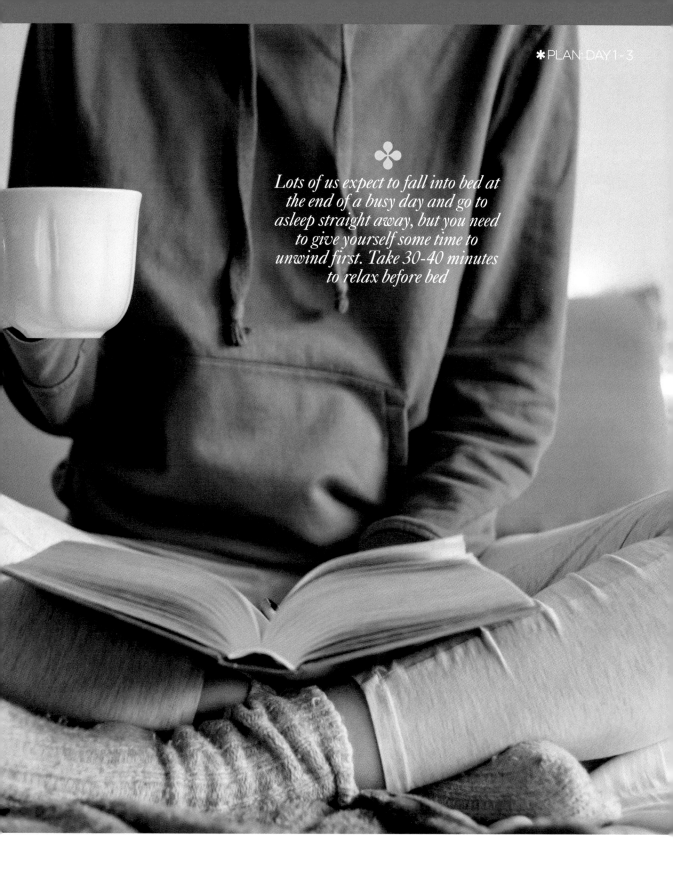

Lots of us expect to fall into bed at the end of a busy day and go to asleep straight away, but you need to give yourself some time to unwind first. Take 30-40 minutes to relax before bed

10
SURPRISING
SLEEP FIXES
to try tonight

Fed up with counting sheep? Here are some new tricks that really work

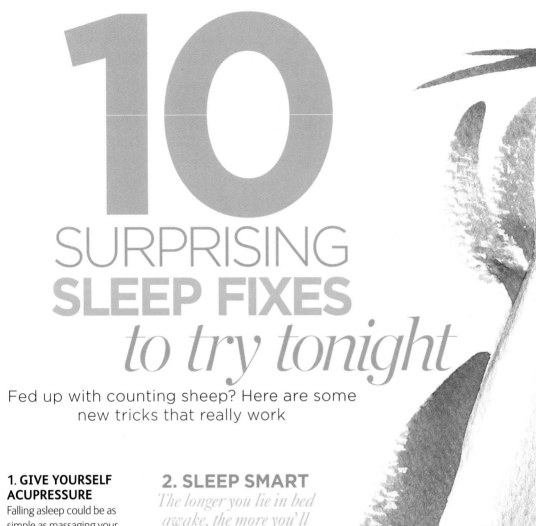

1. GIVE YOURSELF ACUPRESSURE

Falling asleep could be as simple as massaging your wrist. An Italian study found sleep quality improved in 60 per cent of people who massaged an acupuncture point – called the HT7 point – that's linked to anxiety and insomnia. Locate it at the crease where your wrist meets your hand, directly below your little finger. All you need to do is hold your thumb firmly there for two minutes. It busts tension and helps you nod off.

2. SLEEP SMART

The longer you lie in bed awake, the more you'll associate bedtime with feeling anxious. Calculate how long you actually spend asleep and match your time in bed to it. So, if you never fall asleep before 2am, that's the time you should hit the sack. As you feel more relaxed, you can work back to a more normal bedtime.

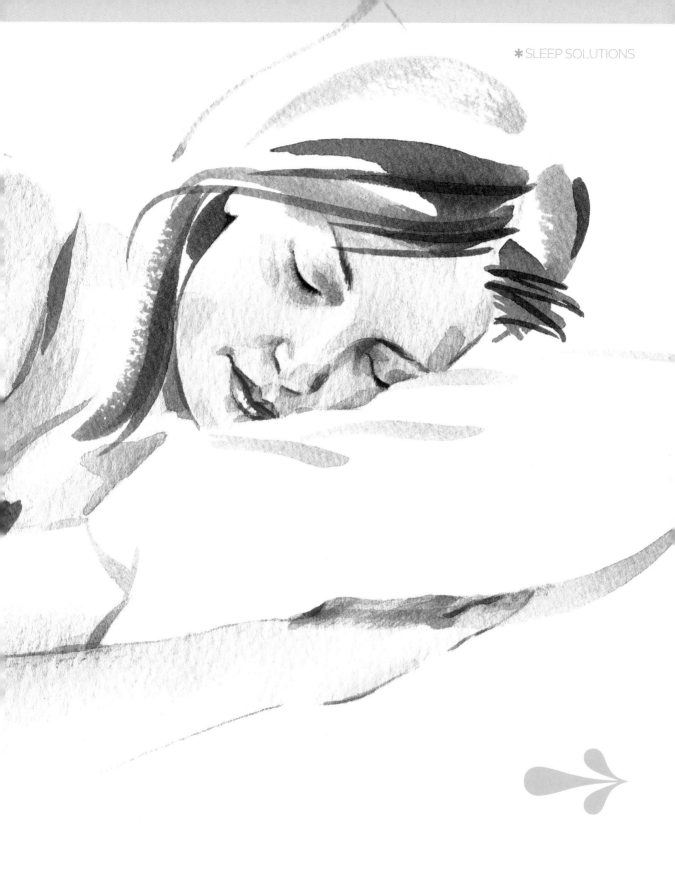

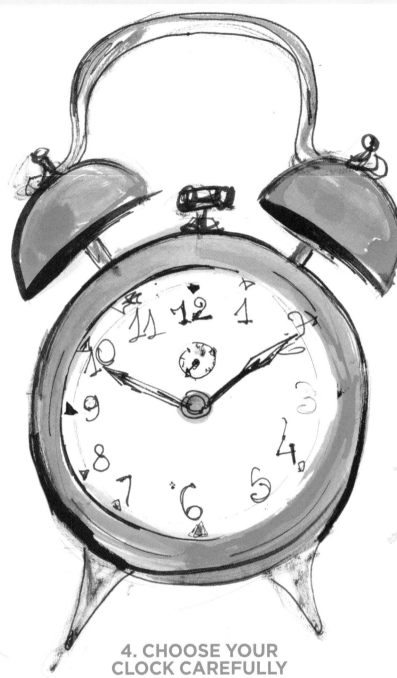

3. FREEZE YOUR PILLOWCASE

Lowering your core body temperature to aid sleep can prove tricky in the summer when nights are usually warmer, which is why you may not sleep so well then or when on holiday. Try this quick trick from sleep expert Dr Nerina Ramlakhan: on hot nights, stick your pillowcase in the freezer for an hour before bed to cool your head and your overall temperature.

4. CHOOSE YOUR CLOCK CAREFULLY

Lots of us now rely on smartphones and tablets to look at the time during the night, or to wake us with an alarm in the morning. But that can mean you get disturbed during the night by the sound of texts, emails and app reminders – and you may feel tempted to look at social media if you wake in the night. Switch off the tech and use a proper alarm clock instead.

5. GET GRATEFUL

Research from Grant MacEwan University, in Canada, has found spending 15 minutes writing in a gratitude journal every evening can transform your sleep. Yes, really – it helps you worry less and feel more optimistic, so you sleep better. Grab a special notebook and list everything you can think of to be grateful for, from your brilliant yoga teacher to the delicious lunch you had with a friend.

6. BREATHE DEEPLY

Holistic expert Dr Andrew Weil has pioneered the 4-7-8 breathing technique to induce a sense of calm and encourage sleep fast – it floods your body with oxygen, which calms you. Here's how to do it. Lightly rest the tip of your tongue just behind your upper teeth and exhale through your mouth, making a whoosh sound. Close your mouth and breathe in through your nose for a count of four. Hold your breath for seven. Exhale through your mouth for eight. Repeat three more times – or until you nod off.

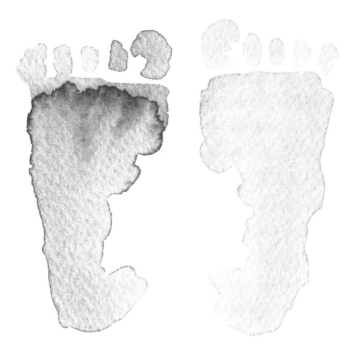

7. ADJUST YOUR DUVET

If you and your partner like different duvet thicknesses, consider switching one double duvet for two singles to make sure you keep your core temperature cool in bed – especially during the summer.

8. WEAR SOCKS TO BED

Keep your tootsies cosy. Warming your feet encourages your blood vessels to dilate, and that sends a signal to the brain that it's time to nod off. It's blood vessel dilation in your extremities – such as in your hands and feet – that is particularly snooze-inducing.

9. TAKE AN ENERGY SUPPLEMENT

Ginseng is often associated with energy rather than sleep but a study from KwanDong University, South Korea, found the herb could actually improve sleep quality and quantity. Take it as a supplement or cut open a capsule and add to a cup of boiling water and honey for a calming bedtime drink.

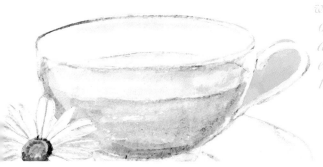

10. LISTEN TO CLASSICAL MUSIC

Studies show listening to classical music for 45 minutes at bedtime can improve sleep in people with insomnia. This kind of music lowers anxiety, distracts your mind and encourages your muscles to relax. Put it on in the background as you get ready for bed.

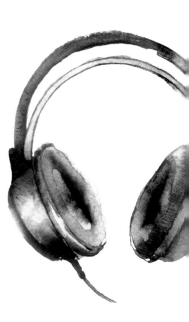

BEAT YOUR
BAD
SLEEP
HABITS

STRUGGLING TO NOD OFF AT NIGHT? IT COULD BE TIME TO TAKE AN INVENTORY OF YOUR PRE-BED ROUTINE – AND IT STARTS EARLIER THAN YOU MIGHT THINK

DAY 4-6

When you lead a busy life with multiple deadlines and spend most of the day multi-tasking, asking your mind to suddenly be quiet enough for you to instantly drop off the moment your head hits the pillow can be a tall order. To maximise your chances of being relaxed enough to sleep, you need to prepare in advance both mentally and physically. Here's what you need to know.

EATING TOO MUCH, TOO LATE

A large, rich meal in the evening isn't the best bedfellow. You won't go to sleep comfortably and may also experience heartburn and indigestion once you lie down, which can wake you. If you have acid reflux, you might even wake up coughing. 'The best thing to go to bed on is a fairly empty stomach,' says nutrition consultant Ian Marber. 'An active digestive system delays deep sleep, although you don't want to wake hungry either. So aim to have your dinner before 8pm if possible and, if sleeplessness is an issue, try eating your main meal at lunchtime and having a lighter supper.' Soup with butter beans stirred through, or chicken or fish with steamed vegetables are good, healthy choices.

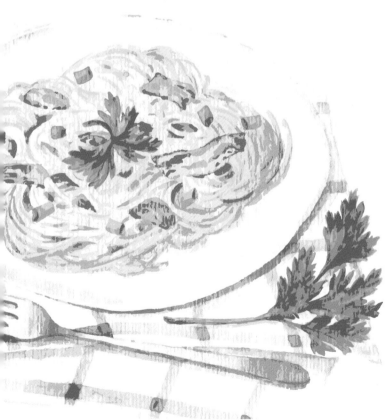

NODDING OFF ON THE SOFA

If you don't get enough sleep at night, you might find your eyes getting heavy during the afternoon or early evening. A short nap (20 minutes or less) can be restorative, but if you snooze for 45-90 minutes, you'll have moved into deep, slow-wave sleep and could wake feeling worse. You'll also be less likely to sleep that evening, so just after lunch is best for short snoozes. 'Avoid naps after 3pm,' says Professor Jim Horne, sleep expert and emeritus professor at Loughborough University. 'It takes longer to drop off at night the more recently you've slept in the day.'

BURNING THE MIDNIGHT OIL

As anyone who works in the evenings knows, it's hard to arrive home from your shift and switch straight off. The same goes if you're working from home, sitting on your laptop until late at night. Ideally, we all need some down time, away from spreadsheets, Word documents or emails. Even if you're on a deadline, decide on a bedtime, set an alarm for 30-60 minutes before that and stop work. Better to get up early and refreshed if you still have tasks to finish off.

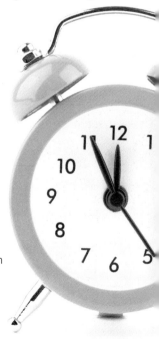

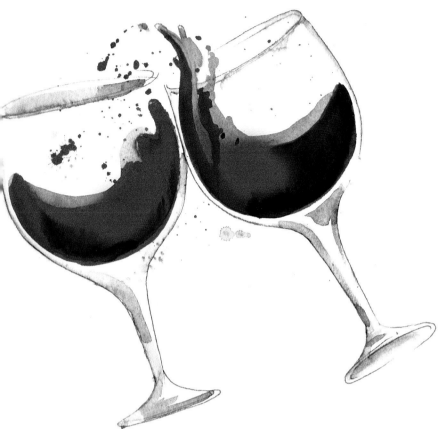

TOO MUCH SCREEN TIME

There's another reason working late keeps you awake – the blue light emitted by your computer suppresses the hormone melatonin, which promotes good quality, deep sleep. The same goes for smartphones, tablets, even your TV. A study at the Brain & Psychological Sciences Institute at Swinburne University of Technology in Australia found using a mobile phone 30 minutes before sleep disrupts the REM phase. And a similar study at the University of Zurich found it altered brain waves, also affecting sleep.

Many devices now come equipped with tools to adjust the colours and brightness of your screen in the evenings (such as Night Shift on iPhone). But better still to shut down all screens for, ideally, two to three hours before bed. Falling asleep to the TV is also a no-no – if you have a TV in your bedroom, move it out for a while and see what the effect is on your sleep.

DRINKING ALCOHOL

They're called nightcaps for a reason and, indeed, a small amount of alcohol can help you drift off. Too much, though and, while you may collapse into what seems like a deep sleep, you're likely to sleep fitfully and wake numerous times as alcohol disrupts the deeper phases of sleep. 'Whether a nightcap or a mug of cocoa is more your style, neither are likely to improve your slumber,' agrees Marber. 'Alcohol may help you get to sleep but, ultimately, disturbs it and, if you're very sensitive, the sugar and caffeine in cocoa won't help. Herbal tea or water is better. But remember not to drink too close to bedtime,' he adds, 'or a full bladder will wake you!' And avoid diuretic herbal teas such as fennel. Valerian and chamomile are both known for their soothing properties so are good choices.

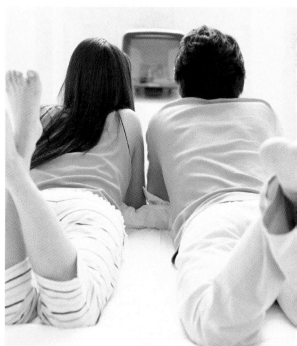

YOUR WEEKEND LIE-INS

We know it's tempting, but try not to lie in for too long. 'Get into the habit of going to bed and rising at the same time, even at weekends,' says Harrold. 'This will help regulate your sleep patterns so you'll soon become sleepy and wake up naturally at the same times each day.' Another reason to avoid lounging in bed at the weekends? Lying in late – which sleep researchers have dubbed 'social jetlag' – has been linked with increased cholesterol and triglycerides, which may increase heart disease risk.

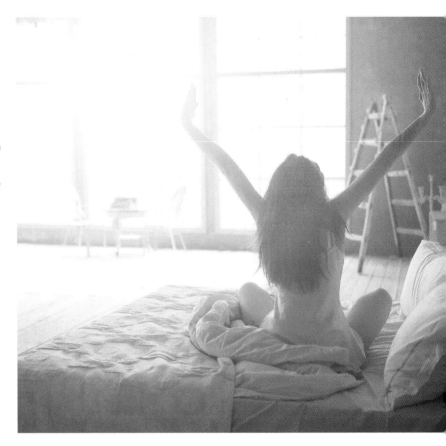

TOO MUCH CAFFEINE

People's sensitivity to caffeine varies wildly. Some people can drink strong coffee night and day and sleep like a log, while others can't have a cuppa after 4pm in case it disrupts their kip. But it's a good rule of thumb for everyone to switch to herbal teas in the evening. And if you're really struggling to sleep, consider quitting caffeine in the afternoons, too. And be aware it's not just in coffee and tea – you'll find this stimulant in cola, energy drinks, green tea, some health supplements (particularly fitness-related), chocolate and all the new, trendy snacks containing raw cacao. Watch out for painkillers, too, if you're particularly sensitive – anything labelled 'express' tends to contain caffeine as it helps your body absorb the painkiller more quickly.

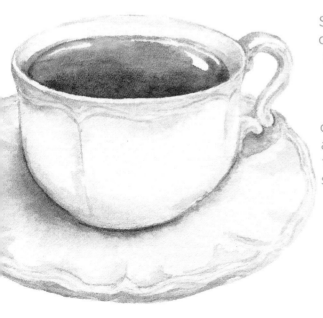

TAKING YOUR TROUBLES TO BED WITH YOU

We've all been there – your body is exhausted but your mind refuses to let you sleep. Maybe you keep replaying a meeting at work in an attempt to better understand why a colleague said what they did, or perhaps you keep thinking of what you should have said to that friend who criticised you for something that wasn't actually your fault. Unfortunately, what your brain is doing by this is keeping you awake, to give you the chance to solve your latest work, relationship or money worry. Your thoughts go round and round in your head, and the longer the answers (and sleep) elude you, the more agitated you become.

Putting in place all the wind-down suggestions above should help, but another tried and tested technique is to keep a notebook by your bed and scribble down a few thoughts to 'park' them for the night. You might want to write down anything that's worrying you. Or perhaps write your to-do list for the next day, so you don't lie down and start mentally compiling it, instead.

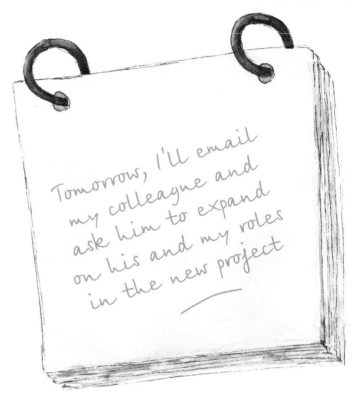

Tomorrow, I'll email my colleague and ask him to expand on his and my roles in the new project

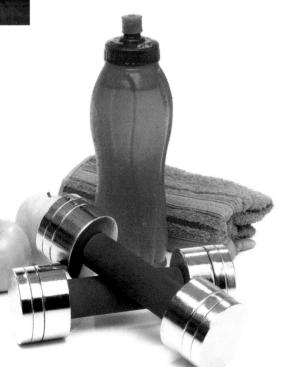

LATE-NIGHT EXERCISE

Keeping active helps promote restful sleep – if you haven't exerted yourself during the day, sleep may elude you at night. 'You lie down and your body says, "what's the point of this? I don't need it",' says independent sleep expert Dr Neil Stanley (thesleepconsultancy.com).

But what if you go to the opposite extreme? If you lead a busy life, it can be tempting to fit in late-night sessions rather than skip them. 'Don't leave it too late, though,' says Stanley. 'Your body temperature rises when you exercise and the subsequent cooling process mimics what happens as your body prepares for sleep. An evening gym session or run may mean you're too stimulated and hot to sleep well.'

Instead, try streaming a relaxing yoga class – see yogaia.com – and flick to page 64 for some simple pre-bed stretches you can try.

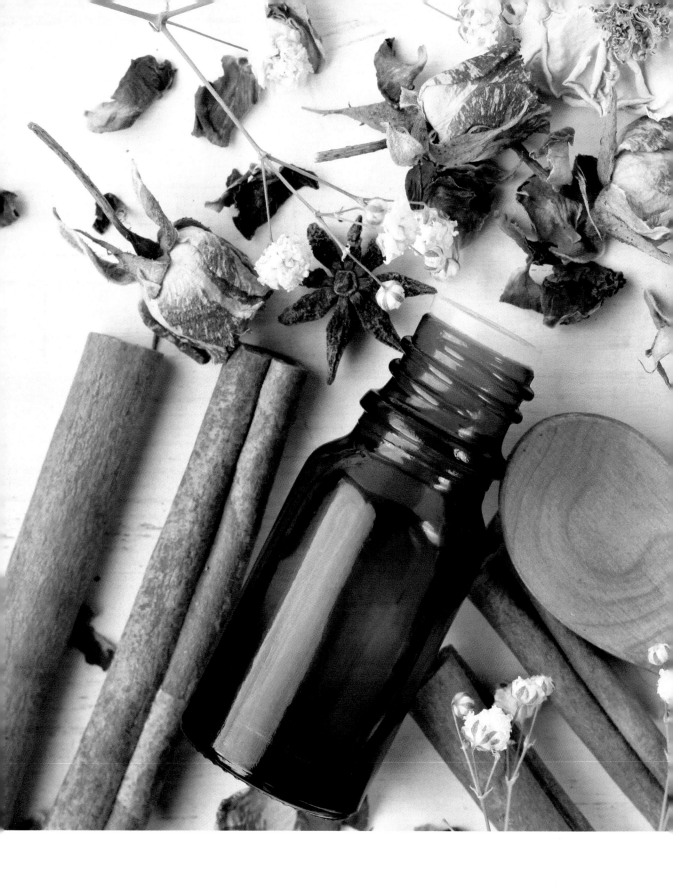

YOUR SLEEP
PRESCRIPTION

Now it's time to delve a bit deeper and start working seriously on getting quality sleep. For most of us, poor sleep is an emotional issue – and tackling your tick-tocking mind is the most important step to nodding off and staying asleep – as you'll discover on p54. Alternative remedies really come into their own when it comes to sleep, and can be a great support – we've rounded up the best, including one you may never have heard of (p50). And start getting to grips with your sleep as soon as you get up – yes, really! – with our guide to the perfect day for a great night's kip (p68).

4

ALTERNATIVE THERAPIES
FOR PERFECT
SLUMBER

Want to avoid sleeping pills? Try these holistic cures

Alternative therapies really come into their own when it comes to improving sleep quality and quantity. If you have long-term sleep issues, you might prefer the idea of a natural approach as opposed to popping pills. And the following therapies can help anyone with poor-quality sleep, not just hardcore insomniacs. Here's our round-up of the best methods to improve your shuteye.

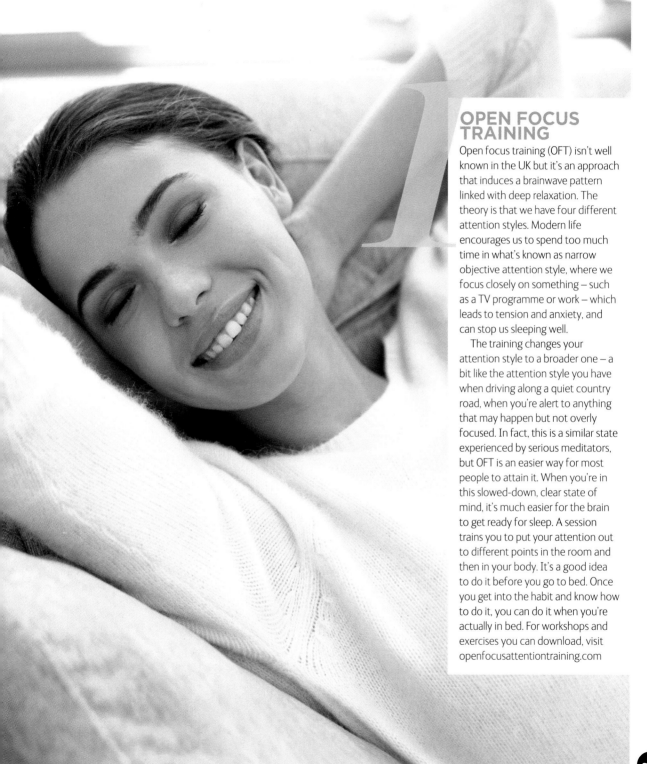

1

OPEN FOCUS TRAINING

Open focus training (OFT) isn't well known in the UK but it's an approach that induces a brainwave pattern linked with deep relaxation. The theory is that we have four different attention styles. Modern life encourages us to spend too much time in what's known as narrow objective attention style, where we focus closely on something – such as a TV programme or work – which leads to tension and anxiety, and can stop us sleeping well.

The training changes your attention style to a broader one – a bit like the attention style you have when driving along a quiet country road, when you're alert to anything that may happen but not overly focused. In fact, this is a similar state experienced by serious meditators, but OFT is an easier way for most people to attain it. When you're in this slowed-down, clear state of mind, it's much easier for the brain to get ready for sleep. A session trains you to put your attention out to different points in the room and then in your body. It's a good idea to do it before you go to bed. Once you get into the habit and know how to do it, you can do it when you're actually in bed. For workshops and exercises you can download, visit openfocusattentiontraining.com

HYPNOTHERAPY

This technique works on your subconscious to induce deep relaxation. Some therapists might take you through guided visualisations, encouraging you to imagine yourself in a beautiful, peaceful place, for example, in a session normally lasting up to an hour. The theory is that when you're in a state of hypnosis, your unconscious mind is open to suggestions of sleep. There isn't a solid bank of evidence behind hypnosis for sleep, but some research has shown hypnotherapy helps improve the deeper phases of sleep, and many insomniacs swear by it. A practitioner will often teach you how to self-hypnotise, and there are also lots of books, CDs, apps and YouTube videos to help you hypnotise yourself – it's often a question of experimenting to find the one that works for you. The British Society of Clinical Hypnosis – bsch.org.uk – can help you find a practitioner that practises near to you.

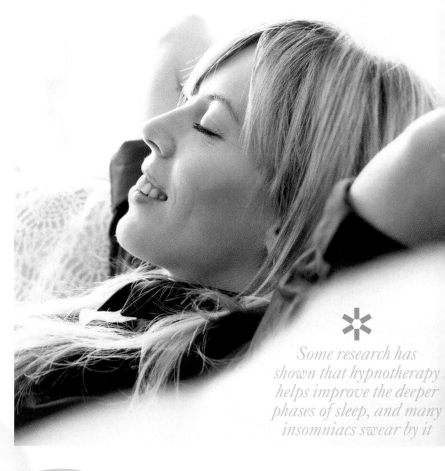

✳

Some research has shown that hypnotherapy helps improve the deeper phases of sleep, and many insomniacs swear by it

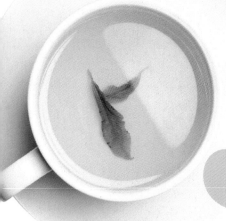

HERBS

Some studies have shown herbal remedies can help improve sleep quality, and may even help those trying to stop taking sleeping pills. Valerian is the main herb that's been studied for its ability to soothe anxiety and ease sleep problems. Herbs aren't a quick fix and won't knock you out like conventional sleeping pills but you'll need to give valerian a chance to work as research shows it may be a few weeks before you notice any changes. Visit a herbal practitioner for a tailored blend to help you. For general relaxation, you could try drinking valerian as a tea before bed. You'll often find it combined in teas and remedies with other traditionally soothing herbs such as hops and passionflower.

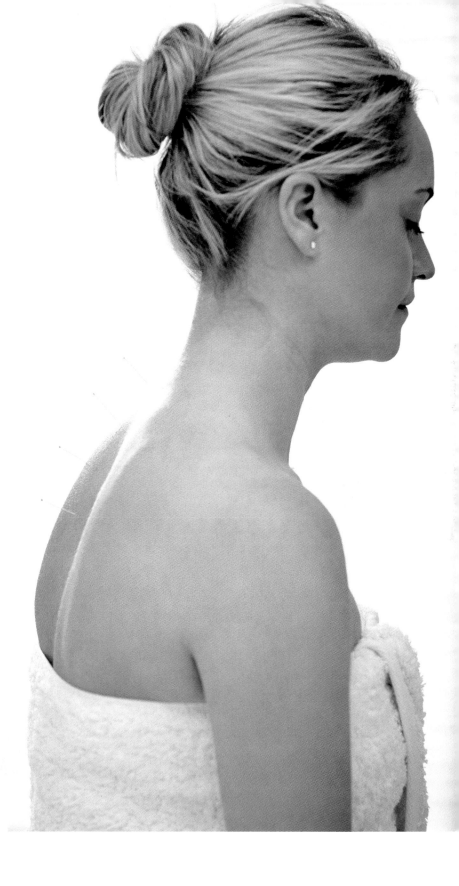

ACUPUNCTURE

Acupuncture – where fine needles are inserted into particular points on the body – is commonly used in China to treat sleep disorders. This ancient Chinese approach may help tackle even long-term insomnia, according to studies. A 2009 analysis of 46 trials looking at acupuncture and insomnia found acupuncture is effective for aiding sleep, although more research is needed.

The traditional theory is that it allows the body's 'chi' energy to flow smoothly, which increases your sense of relaxation. In Western thinking, it's thought to induce sleepiness by having an effect on the central nervous system. Some research has suggested stimulating certain points linked to areas of the brain thought to reduce sensitivity to pain and stress can help. Needling these points also helps by encouraging relaxation and deactivating the overthinking, analytical brain, which often keeps you awake.

In a session, you'll lie down and have needles inserted into points on your body believed to be connected to insomnia, for example, the inner wrists. The needles are usually inserted very superficially so it shouldn't be painful. However, if you have 'blocked chi', you may experience a stronger sensation, although this usually dies down after a few moments. You'll then be left to lie down, usually for about 30 minutes. You would normally have a course of several acupuncture treatments, although the exact number depends on your particular issues. Visit acupuncture.org.uk to find a practitioner near you.

CALM
YOUR
MIND

DOES ANXIETY OR A BUSY BRAIN KEEP YOU AWAKE AT NIGHT? TRY THESE EASY, PROVEN SOLUTIONS

DAY 7-9

Whether you have long-term insomnia or you just struggle with poor sleep from time to time, soothing your mind is crucial. When you're stressed, your brain senses danger and remains on alert, which means it keeps you awake. If sleep is stressing you out, the following psychological techniques have been shown to help switch off your mind and lull you into shuteye. Plus, we have some simple relaxation tricks to help you unwind every night.

LEARN CBT

Cognitive behavioural therapy (CBT) is the gold standard treatment for stress and anxiety, and it has also been shown to help improve sleep. It teaches you techniques to deal with the thoughts that keep you awake at night, while also helping you to rebuild a new, healthy sleep schedule. You'll also learn ways to help you cope generally with stress.

CBT is particularly useful when you've developed primary insomnia – in other words, when your inability to sleep is caused by worry about not sleeping. It teaches you to challenge thoughts such as, 'I won't be able to cope with work if I don't sleep' or 'I'll look terrible for my date tomorrow if I'm tired', and replace them with more rational thoughts such as, 'I'll be tired tomorrow but I've coped before' or 'I might not feel my best but it's unlikely anyone else will be able to tell'.

You may also learn relaxation techniques and sleep restriction – working out how many hours you actually spend asleep, and only going to bed for those hours, even if that means you stay up until the early hours of the morning so you gradually wind back to a normal bedtime. Clinical trials have shown that, on average, 70 per cent of people with even serious long-term sleep problems get lasting benefits from CBT.

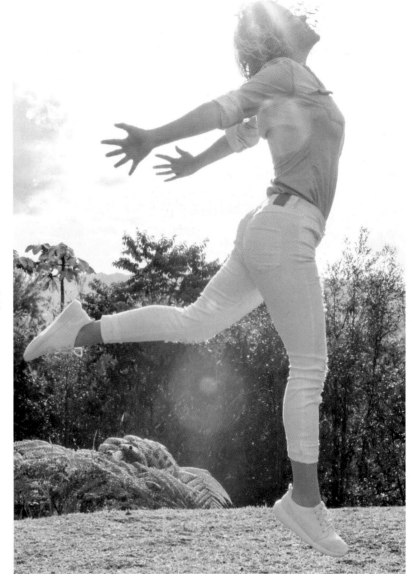

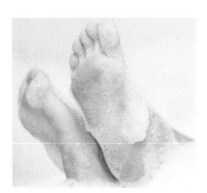

TRY IT NOW: Jot down a worry you have about sleeping tonight. For example, you might write down that you woke at 3am last night, and you're afraid you're going to do the same tonight, and you're worried that you won't be able to cope tomorrow if you're tired. Then think about this thought – can you be sure it's true? Just because you woke last night does that mean you will wake again tonight? Perhaps you can think about other times you've woken in the early hours and still managed to nod off after, or cope the following day. Ask yourself how much it will really matter if you don't get as much sleep as you want. And think about what practical steps you can take to ease your stress before you go to bed. Would a relaxing bath help, for example?

DO SOMETHING SIMPLE

Colouring in is a great pre-bed activity to prepare your mind for sleep, says Dr Nerina Ramlakhan, sleep expert for Silentnight. co.uk 'It slows the mind down, taking your brain from the stimulated beta mode into the alpha-theta states that are almost meditative.' Or do another mindful activity – something that requires concentration but not too much active thinking, such as a dot-to-dot puzzle, ironing, baking or simple sewing.

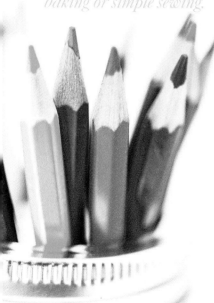

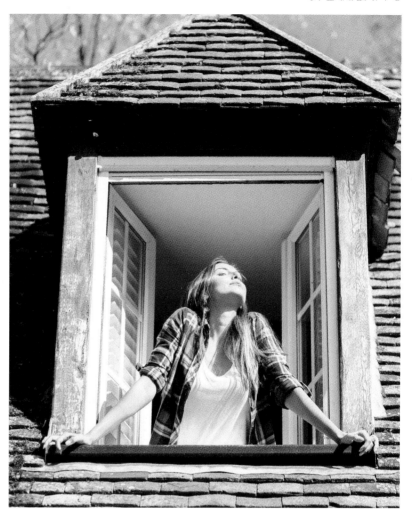

TAKE BREAKS DURING THE DAY

It's not just before bed that you need to unwind. 'Pushing on through a stressful day can overstimulate your central nervous system and give you that "tired but wired" feeling that can make it harder to fall asleep later,' says Ramlakhan. She advises disciplining yourself into taking a three- to five-minute break every 90 minutes. Move away from your desk, walk around the block, go and make a cup of tea. This will help you wind down more easily in the evening.

While psychological therapies can help in the longer term, don't underestimate the power of simple relaxation techniques.

GO FOR ACT THERAPY

Another technique to try is acceptance and commitment therapy (ACT), a strategy that has its origins in CBT. But rather than helping you change the way you think and feel, ACT aims to change your relationship with your thoughts and feelings. This is a subtle difference but Dr Guy Meadows of The Sleep School considers it a superior method for dealing with insomnia. 'Sometimes, challenging negative thinking can actually increase anxiety which, ironically, leads to wakefulness,' he says. If you take a 'don't fight it, feel it' approach, you may find it easier to relax.

Instead of fighting anxious thoughts or trying to change them, in ACT you try simply noticing the thoughts and even being a little playful with them. For example, you could try thanking that worrying thought for turning up again, then turn your attention to your breath, feeling the air pass through your nostrils, your chest rising and falling, your until your brain realises it doesn't have to stay alert and allows you to relax and nod off. Essentially, your brain gets 'bored' and switches off. Accepting anxious thoughts takes practice but, ultimately, induces relaxation, so the brain learns there's nothing to be worried about and allows you to sleep. Visit thesleepschool.org for courses and workshops.

TRY IT NOW: 'Instead of worrying about how little sleep you've had or how bad the next day will be, use a simple mindfulness exercise to keep yourself in the present,' says Meadows. One good way to do this is to focus on your sense of touch, he says. Ask yourself, 'What can I feel right now? For example, you might say to yourself that you can feel the duvet on your toes, the mattress against your body, the pillow on your face.' Focusing on the here and now will stop you going into panic mode.

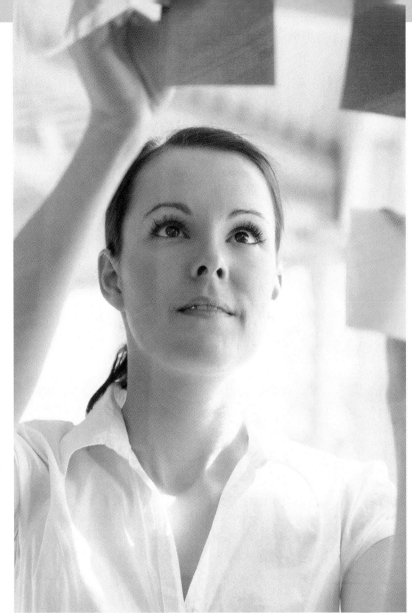

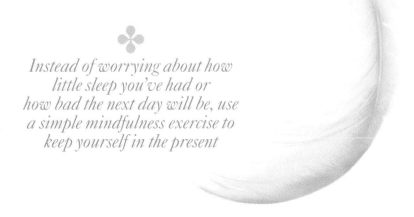

Instead of worrying about how little sleep you've had or how bad the next day will be, use a simple mindfulness exercise to keep yourself in the present

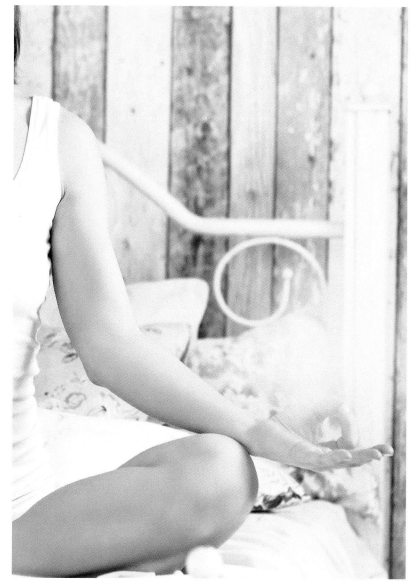

GET MEDITATING

It doesn't matter if you've never been able to master any traditional meditation techniques – it's about finding your own way to clear your mind. Do whatever works for you. Calm, even breathing is key as it will naturally slow your heart rate, and, if you lengthen the exhale, you will automatically stimulate your rest and relax response. As you breathe in, say: 'I am breathing in' and as you breathe out, say: 'I am breathing out'. This anchors you in the present. You could also focus on taking your attention to different body parts, say your skin surface, travelling from your feet to your head. Or find a visualisation exercise on the internet and follow that. Don't put too much pressure on yourself – even having five minutes to quieten your mind makes a difference. If you try to meditate for too long before you're experienced at it, you might end up getting frustrated. Start small.

GO OUTSIDE

Spending time outdoors in nature, particularly in green spaces or near water, has been shown to help relax your mind and bust stress. So it's a good idea to head outdoors during the day, even if it's just for a 15-minute stroll. If you can go for a walk with friends, so much the better – other research has found walking in a group is the ultimate tension-blitzer.

ESSENTIAL
HELPERS

**Use these relaxing aromatherapy blends
to ease you into a good night's rest**

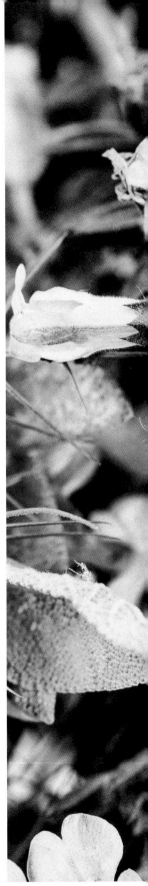

Calming and soothing essential oils have been used for generations to promote relaxation and sleep. Whether you place a cotton ball or tissue infused with relaxing oils near your pillow, add them to your bath water or diffuser an hour before bedtime, or gently massage your feet and legs with a soothing blend in the evening, the quieting properties of certain oils can help you drift off to a into a super-restorative slumber.

But while sniffing the right oils can help you get the rest you need, you do need to exercise some caution. Essential oils are powerful things. Even a few drops can be enough to fragrance a large room and an over-scented space can have the opposite of a soporific effect.

Making your own blend is easy and affordable. Stick to sleep-promoting essential oils such as Roman chamomile, clary sage and bergamot. Lavender oil is famous for its sedative properties – a study in the journal *Perceptual & Motor Skills* showed it to improve the mean sleep scores of participants – but more than three drops in a blend can actually be stimulating, so don't be tempted to add more than a couple of drops if making your own blend. Be sure to avoid known energising oils such as cypress, rosemary, grapefruit, lemon and peppermint.

Here are some recipes to try – they can all can be adapted. For example, the bath blend can just as easily be a massage oil – simply leave out the Epsom salts and add an ounce of carrier oil instead. Only use one blend at a time, though, even if you decide to bathe in and diffuse oils on the same evening. You don't want to overwhelm your senses before bedtime, even with calming combinations!

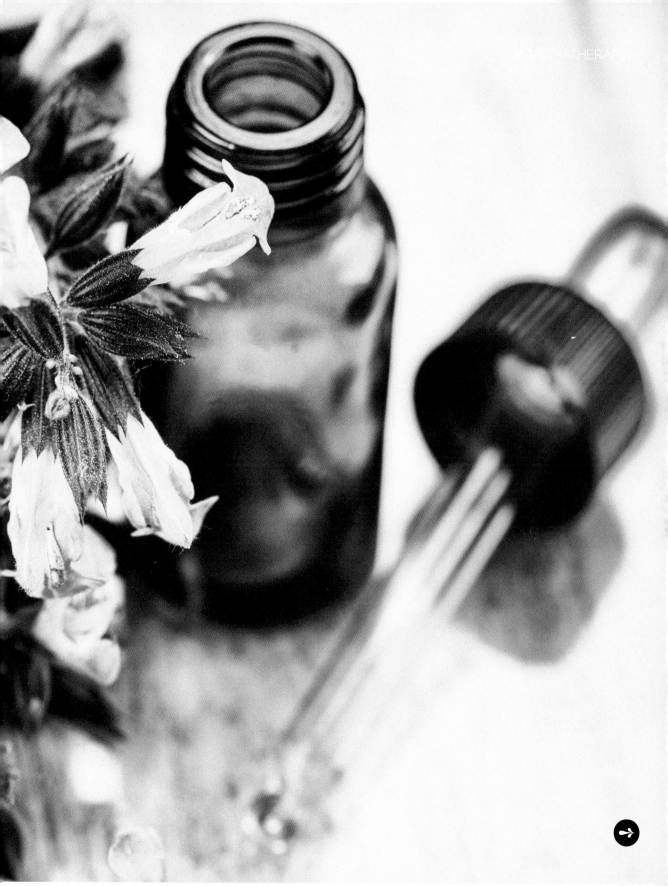

Bath blend

'A relaxing bath is the best way to unwind after a hectic day, but what's even better is enhancing the experience with essential oils handpicked for your mood and needs,' says Nawsheen Goolamally, senior spa therapist at Marshall Street Spa, managed by Everyone Active (everyoneactive.com). Here's her recipe for a calming bath blend:

- 2-3 drops lavender oil
- 1 tbsp jojoba oil
- 2 drops geranium oil
- 2-3 drops chamomile
- 5 drops clary sage oil
- Handful Epsom salts

Sleep mist

'One of the best and most surprising tips I've found for sleeping better is to stretch for 10 to 30 minutes before bed,' says Nawsheen. 'A relaxing pillow mist can also help you drift off.'

- A tiny funnel
- A mist bottle
- Distilled water
- 15 drops wild orange oil
- 10-15 drops chamomile oil
- 20 drops lavender oil

Use the funnel to add all your essential oils to the bottle, then fill the rest with distilled water. Shake before each use. If you want a much stronger scent, you can always add more drops, but I suggest starting with these. This can be used every day. Spritz a spray or two on your pillows, sheets and/or pyjamas before bed.

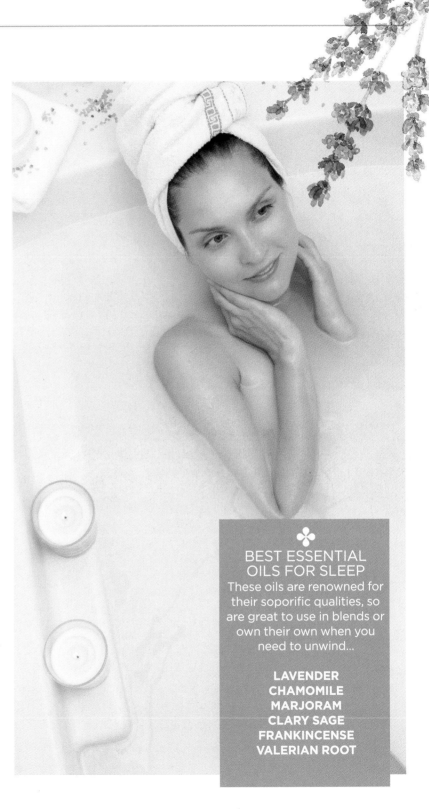

❖

BEST ESSENTIAL OILS FOR SLEEP

These oils are renowned for their soporific qualities, so are great to use in blends or own their own when you need to unwind...

**LAVENDER
CHAMOMILE
MARJORAM
CLARY SAGE
FRANKINCENSE
VALERIAN ROOT**

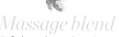

Massage blend

- 2 drops lavender oil
- 2 drops tangerine oil
- 2 drops sweet orange oil
- 2 drops chamomile oil
- 2 drops ylang ylang oil
- 2 drops marjoram oil
- 1 oz carrier oil

Blend the oils well in a clean dark-coloured glass bottle and work the mixture into your body using gentle massage movements wherever you feel you have tension or your muscles ache, to help you ease yourself into a restful state. Massage your feet, legs, tummy, chest, lower back, shoulders and/or upper arms an hour before you go to bed – or if you can find a willing friend to do it, all the better!

Pillow blend

- 8 drops lavender oil
- 5 drops vetiver oil
- 5 drops sweet orange oil

Blend the oils well in a clean dark-coloured glass bottle. Add one or two drops to a tissue and place inside your pillowcase to help you fall into a deep sleep. Be careful where you place the tissue, though. The essential oils shouldn't come into direct contact with your face or skin as you sleep, so ensure the tissue is tucked away.

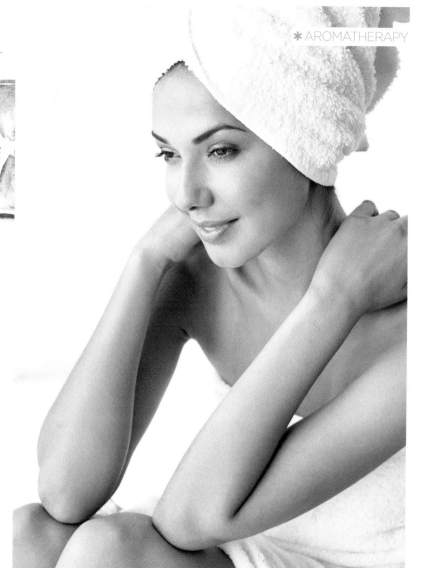

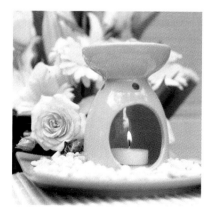

Diffuser blend

- 2 drops Roman chamomile oil
- 1 drop clary sage oil
- 1 drop bergamot oil

This powerful blend can help you switch off at the end of a hectic day. Apply the drops to your diffuser to fragrance your room with a sleep-inducing aroma before bedtime.

To use these oils as a pillow blend, adjust the quantities to:

- 10 drops Roman chamomile oil
- 5 drops clary sage oil
- 5 drops bergamot oil

Blend the oils and use as guided in the Pillow blend above.

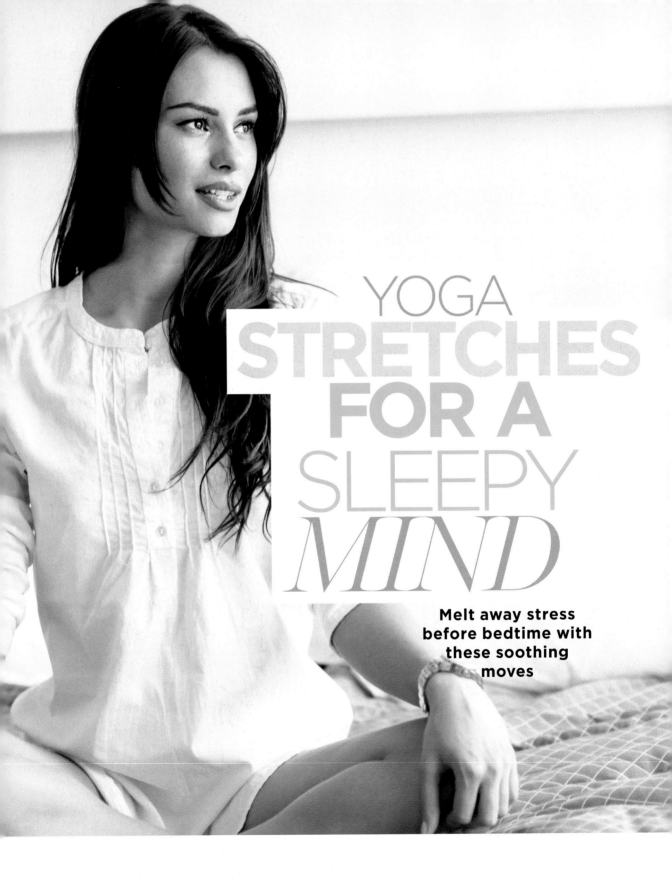

YOGA
STRETCHES
FOR A
SLEEPY
MIND

**Melt away stress
before bedtime with
these soothing
moves**

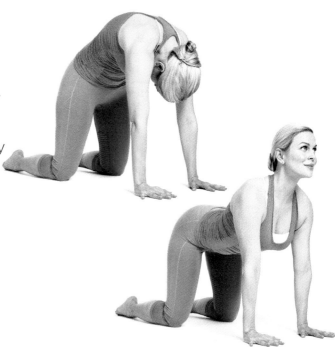

We all hold a lot of tension in our bodies, believes yoga teacher Hassan (h2yoga.info). 'Doing some simple yoga poses before bed can really help you unwind and have a deeper sleep. Poses from yin yoga – a slow, restorative form – are especially relaxing. Or try the following poses in the half hour before you go to bed. Hold each for 10 to 15 breaths.

1 CHILD'S POSE

Kneel on the floor. Touch your big toes together and sit on your heels, then exhale and lay your body down flat over your thighs. Try to broaden your sacrum across the back of your pelvis and lengthen your tailbone towards your heels while you lift the base of your skull away from the back of your neck. If you feel more comfortable, you could also try this pose with your knees hip-width apart, leaving your toes touching. Breathe deeply into the back of your body.

2 CAT-COW

This is made up of two poses flowing into each other. Start with cat pose. Begin on your hands and knees with your back flat, your knees directly below your hips and your wrists, elbows and shoulders in line and perpendicular to the floor. Hold your head in a neutral position, eyes looking at the floor. Exhale and round your spine towards the ceiling, like a cat stretching. Keep your knees and shoulders in position. Release your head towards the floor. As you inhale, come back to your neutral tabletop position then lift your sitting bones and chest towards the ceiling, allowing your belly to sink toward the floor. Lift your head to look straight ahead or upwards – this is the cow element of the pose. Keep flowing between the two.

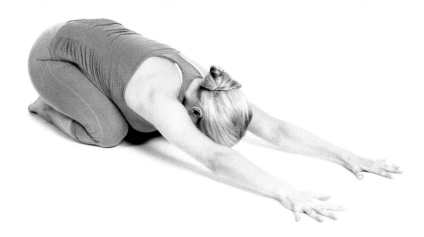

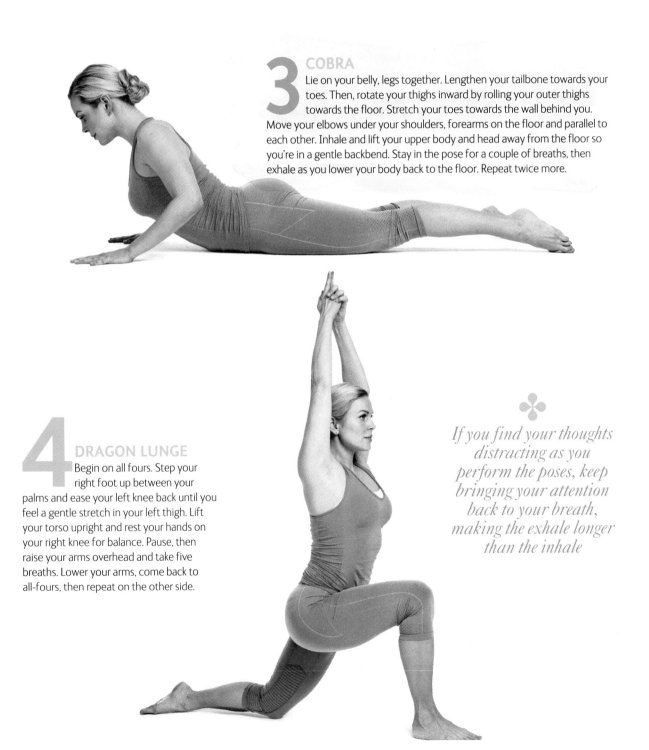

3 COBRA

Lie on your belly, legs together. Lengthen your tailbone towards your toes. Then, rotate your thighs inward by rolling your outer thighs towards the floor. Stretch your toes towards the wall behind you. Move your elbows under your shoulders, forearms on the floor and parallel to each other. Inhale and lift your upper body and head away from the floor so you're in a gentle backbend. Stay in the pose for a couple of breaths, then exhale as you lower your body back to the floor. Repeat twice more.

4 DRAGON LUNGE

Begin on all fours. Step your right foot up between your palms and ease your left knee back until you feel a gentle stretch in your left thigh. Lift your torso upright and rest your hands on your right knee for balance. Pause, then raise your arms overhead and take five breaths. Lower your arms, come back to all-fours, then repeat on the other side.

If you find your thoughts distracting as you perform the poses, keep bringing your attention back to your breath, making the exhale longer than the inhale

5 RELAXED DOWNWARD DOG

Start on your hands and knees, with knees directly under your hips. Keep your hands shoulder-width apart. Your wrists should be slightly in front of your shoulders. Let your index fingers point straight ahead. Press down through your hands, especially through the thumb and index finger. Engage your lower belly and draw it in – think about scooping your lower belly up along your spine. Tuck your toes in and lift your hips up. Pedal through your feet a few times. Don't worry about trying to get your heels onto the floor – this is a more relaxed version of downward dog.

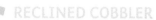

6 RECLINED COBBLER

Start in a seated position with your legs straight out in front of you. Gently pull your knees towards your body and bring the soles of your feet together, then let your thighs fall open. Draw your heels towards your pelvis. Now lie down, over a bolster or pillow if you are able, with your arms alongside your body, palms turned up. Keep your shoulders relaxed. Make sure your body is soft, with no strain anywhere. Don't worry about pushing your knees down further to the ground – just let them fall out as far as they can comfortably, using cushions or blocks to support them if that feels more comfortable for your groins.

YOUR
SLEEP
FRIENDLY
DAY

GETTING A GOOD NIGHT'S KIP
ISN'T JUST ABOUT WHAT YOU
DO AT BEDTIME. FOR THE BEST
CHANCE OF A STRESS-FREE
SLUMBER, TRY THIS TIMETABLE
AND SEE THE DIFFERENCE
IT MAKES...

DAY 10-12

If you want to optimise your chances of peaceful sleep, what you choose to do not just in the hour or two before bed but throughout the day can have a major impact on the quality of your kip. Here we show you the routines, food choices, exercises and mindful living that prep your body for deeper relaxation and readiness for sleep. As you become familiar with the techniques, notice which ones really make a difference to your mood and energy, and focus on those when time is short.

7:00 WAKE NATURALLY

Swap your normal bedside lamp and noisy alarm for a daylight-simulating device, such as the Lumie Bodyclock Iris 500 (£160; lumie.com). Its soothing light fades like a sunset as you drift off or read in bed, prompting your body to start producing the sleep hormone melatonin. By morning, instead of a loud 'beep beep' to shock you out of deep sleep, the lamp gradually brightens to wake you like a sunrise. It also features two diffusion chambers that safely heat essential oils, so you can sleep to the scent of soporific lavender and wake to zingy lemon (or the essential oil of your choice).

7:10 LET THE LIGHT IN

As soon as you're on your feet, walk around your home opening curtains and blinds and letting in as much natural light as you can. Experts say this really helps dispel that 'sleep inertia' grogginess and re-energises you. If it's still dark outside, aim to get out in daylight as soon as it dawns.

7:05 COMPLETE A SLEEP DIARY

Keep a notebook and pen by your bed and take a moment each morning to note down how you slept in the night. 'This will highlight your particular sleep patterns,' says clinical hypnotherapist Glenn Harrold, author of *Sleep Well Every Night* (Orion, £9.99). 'Note the time you went to bed, to sleep, the total time slept, if you woke, what you did, any remedies you took, the last time you ate or drank, and your moods on going to bed and waking, and so on. After a few weeks, you'll spot the factors that help or hinder your sleep.'

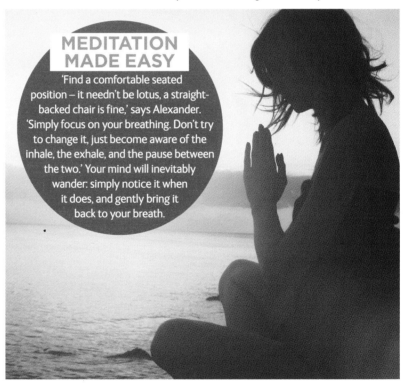

MEDITATION MADE EASY
'Find a comfortable seated position – it needn't be lotus, a straight-backed chair is fine,' says Alexander. 'Simply focus on your breathing. Don't try to change it, just become aware of the inhale, the exhale, and the pause between the two.' Your mind will inevitably wander: simply notice it when it does, and gently bring it back to your breath.

7:15 MAKE TIME FOR MEDITATION

Anxiety can be a big cause of sleeplessness, and there's lots of evidence that regular meditation can help to ease it. Rather than wait until the end of the day when you're feeling stressed and frazzled, aim for a few minutes' meditation first thing, and you'll set yourself up for a calmer, easier day.

'Researchers at UCLA found that mindfulness meditation was as effective as clinical sleep therapy or sleeping pills,' says holistic health expert Jane Alexander, author of *Wellbeing and Mindfulness* (Carlton, £18.99). These days there are lots of apps that guide you through simple meditations – see page 110 for our recommendations. You could learn techniques at a local meditation or yoga class. Or have a go on your own. It needn't be complicated.

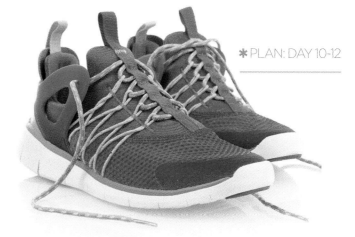

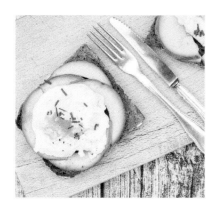

7:30 HAVE BREAKFAST

'Steer clear of carb-heavy breakfasts that might make you sleepy by mid-morning,' warns nutritionist Amanda Hamilton, co-author of gut-health book 'The G Plan Diet (Aster, £8.99). 'Sugary cereals, pastries or toast laden with jam won't keep you full for long. Instead, choose a mix of protein and slow-release carbohydrates, such as wholegrains. 'Something like porridge and seeds made with almond milk would be a filling choice that's easy on your digestion. Or eggs, spinach and avocado on a small slice of sourdough bread. Fruit gets a bad rap these days, but it's a rich source of vitamins.'

8:00 BUILD EXERCISE INTO YOUR COMMUTE

Incorporating activity into your day better prepares your body for rest at night. Try to be more active generally, rather than saving it all up for one intense workout, then sitting in your car or on the bus, at a desk or on the sofa the rest of the time. Your morning commute is the ideal time to start. Could you walk, jog or cycle all or part of it? Even getting off the bus or train a stop or two early, or parking further away from the office is good. Or go for a walk or run at lunchtime.
At home all day? Invest in an activity tracker and aim to get 10,000 steps at day (at least), which may mean a brisk walk around the block morning, mid-day and tea time. You'll feel more energised and alert, as a result.

13:00 RECLAIM YOUR LUNCH BREAK

Forget working through lunch or popping out for a sandwich and shoving it down at your desk. Take time out for lunch, leave your workplace and get outside into the light and fresh air. If you're meeting a friend or colleague, why not go for a walk rather than sit in a café? Or hit the gym for a 30-minute swim or a quick class. Even if you only have a short break, find the time and place to eat slowly and mindfully, returning to your desk nourished and re-energised. 'Make sure you include some protein and wholegrains,' adds Hamilton. 'A salad with quinoa and chicken, fish or tofu would be a good choice.'

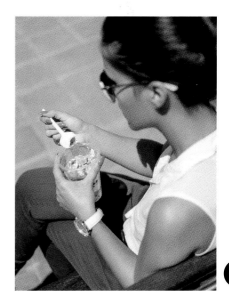

18:00 DO A POST-WORK WORKOUT

If you're heading to the gym, a class or out for a run, early evening is better than late (see Beat your bad sleep habits, page 42). Or it may suit you better to exercise before work or at lunchtime. Keep notes in your sleep diary and you'll soon find the pattern that works best for you. Intense activity such as Spinning or HIIT classes may be best for mornings, and a jog or yoga class for evenings. Or you may find you sleep better after a hard workout early evening – we're all different so mix it up and find what works for you.

20:00 PREPARE FOR TOMORROW

Do you go to bed with your to-do list whirring through your mind? Or spend half an hour in a sleepy fog in the morning, trying to pick out what to wear? Just 10 minutes of simple preparation can put an end to both scenarios. Before you start your bedtime wind-down, choose tomorrow's outfit – yes, including your underwear, tights and shoes – and hang it up in your bedroom. Then get your bag ready with everything you need. If you take lunch to work, prep it now, and put out your breakfast utensils in the kitchen.

19:00 MAKE A LIGHT, BUT NUTRITIOUS, DINNER

For most people, it's better not to eat too late or too much. So keep it light and avoid anything too rich or spicy – you don't want to disrupt sleep with heartburn or a gurgling tummy. 'Some foods contain the amino acid tryptophan,' says Hamilton. 'This converts to the feelgood chemical serotonin in the brain, which then becomes melatonin by night. You'll find tryptophan in turkey, chicken, some seeds, bananas, pulses and milk.'

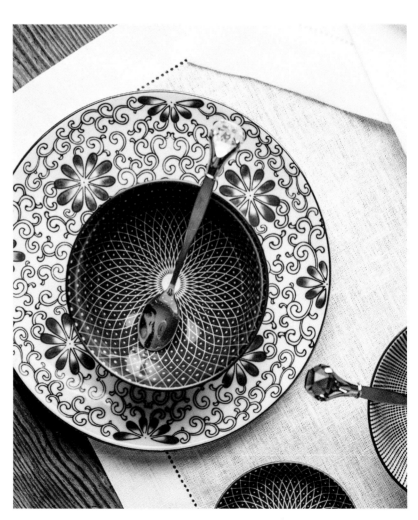

20:15 START YOUR WIND-DOWN EARLY

Turn off all your gadgets a couple of hours before you plan to hit the sack. As we saw in 10 surprising sleep fixes (page 38), the blue light that tech emits interferes with melatonin production. Plus, switching between email, Twitter, Facebook, Instagram and the web is a sure-fire way to keep your brain wired into the night. Some TV is fine if it helps you to decompress from your day, but resist split-screening and put the tech away.

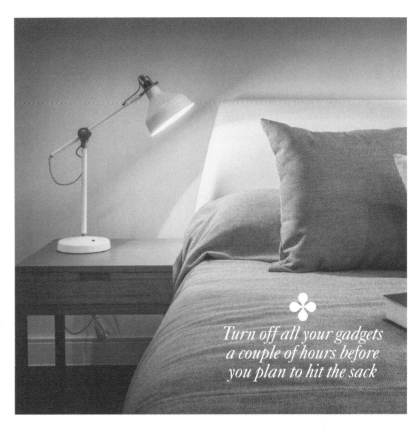

Turn off all your gadgets a couple of hours before you plan to hit the sack

20:30 RUN A BATH

It's a traditional relaxation technique and for good reason. Sinking into a warm bath is wonderfully soothing; not only does it help calm a busy mind, it releases tight muscles and can ease headaches. The gentle raising of your body temperature also triggers your sleep mechanism, according to The Sleep Council. The mineral magnesium is a natural relaxant and studies have shown it is better absorbed through your skin than orally. So, next time you have a bath, add a couple of handfuls of magnesium flakes for an extra blissful soak. They're good after exercise or illness, if you have aches and pains, and can help ease cramps.

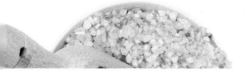

21:45 PREPARE YOUR ROOM

According to Lisa Artis of The Sleep Council, 'In order to get a restful night's sleep you need the right setting, which means a clean, peaceful and welcoming room'. Take a few moments to ensure yours feels cosy and inviting, remembering the 'cool, dark and quiet' rule (see Your sleep hygiene makeover, p32). So, turn the heating down or off, draw the curtains, dim the lights and close the door to minimise noise (such as a washing machine whirring or TV blaring) that may be coming from elsewhere in your home. Tidy away any clutter so your bedroom is the haven you want to retreat to at the end of the day.

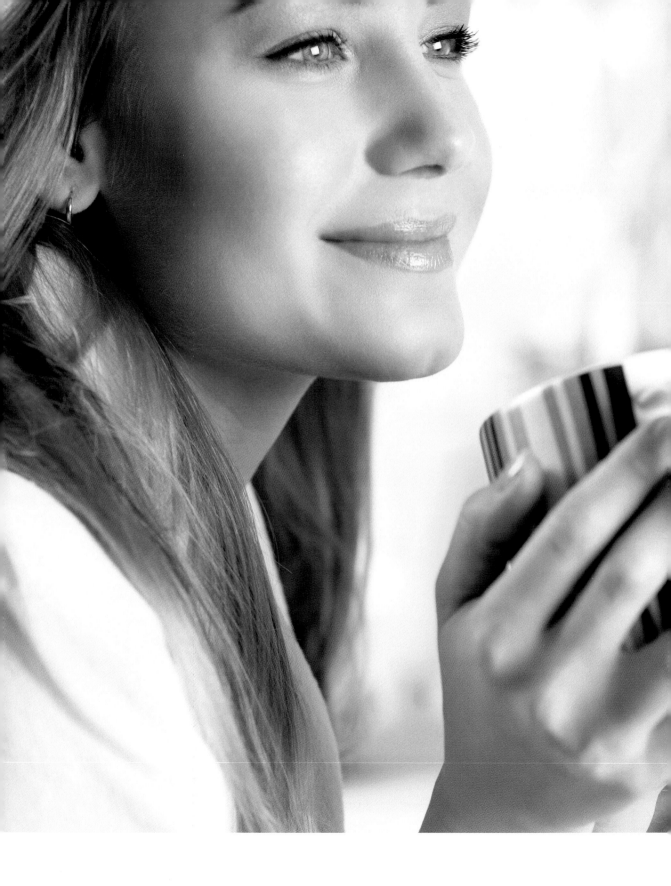

SUPPLEMENTS FOR *GOOD SLEEP*

Nutritional supplements can help you nod off. Here's what to look for...

Contemplating the sheer volume of sleep supplements on offer in any health food shop can be enough to bring on a bout of insomnia. Still, if you choose the right product, it could help you drift off to a decent night's sleep.

While the side effects of prescription sleeping tablets are well known (see page 73), over-the-counter (OTC) sleep-aid medicines sold in pharmacies can also be problematic. That's because they're usually a type of antihistamine that causes morning drowsiness, making activities such as driving and operating machinery dangerous.

Herbal and nutritional supplements can help you sleep without the downsides of prescription or OTC sleeping pills, so look for a product containing the ingredients below to set yourself up for a good night's kip...

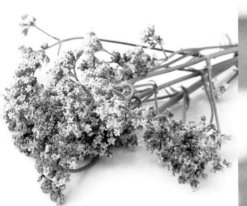

VALERIAN

A traditional herbal medicinal product used for the temporary relief of sleep disturbances, valerian root is also believed to ease the symptoms of mild anxiety. No single compound in valerian has so far been identified as the active sedative agent, but experts believe taking the herb may increase the amount of GABA (gamma-aminobutyric acid), a compound in the brain that activates the major calming neurotransmitters, promoting relaxation and reducing anxiety. Valerian seems to be especially effective when it is combined with hops, according to a 2007 study. A.Vogel Dormeasan Valerian & Hops tincture (£4.15 for 15ml; avogel.co.uk) fits the bill perfectly.

THEANINE

An amino acid derivative found in green tea, theanine has long been known to trigger the release in the brain of GABA. Although GABA supplements are easy to get hold of, the body has difficulty absorbing synthesised GABA. That's why experts tend to recommend supplementing with theanine instead, which the body can easily absorb and, ultimately, use to boost levels of GABA. Nature's Best Pure L-Theanine 200mg (£9.95 for 60 tablets; naturesbest.co.uk) is made to pharmaceutical GMP standards. Experts recommend you never exceed a dose of 600mg to aid sleep.

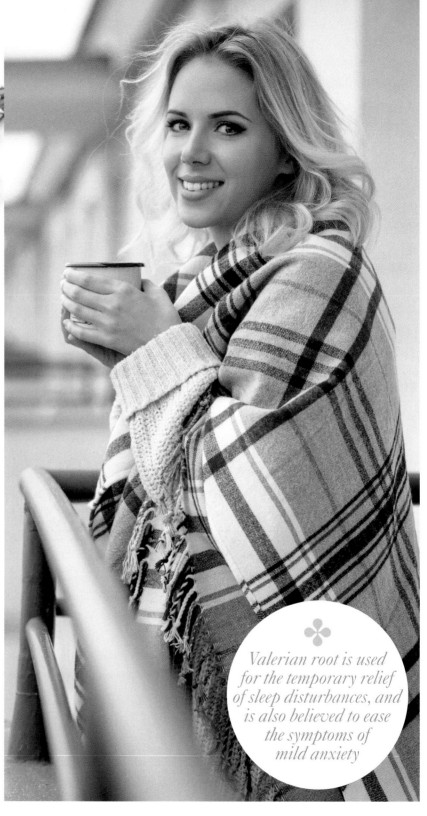

Valerian root is used for the temporary relief of sleep disturbances, and is also believed to ease the symptoms of mild anxiety

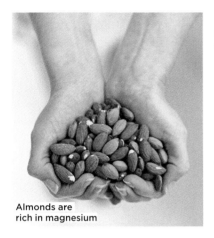

Almonds are
rich in magnesium

5HTP

A precursor to serotonin, the
neurotransmitter that's essential for a
good night's sleep, 5HTP also is used to
enhance mood and decrease appetite.
This amino acid, 5-hydroxytryptophan to
give it its full name, is also a precursor to
melatonin, a hormone that regulates the
normal sleep/wake cycle and is naturally
produced by the body after the sun goes
down, letting us know it's time to fall
asleep (see right). The quality supplement
Higher Nature Serotone 5HTP 100mg
(£12.10 for 30, highernature.co.uk) also
contains specific co-factor B vitamins
and zinc to support the nervous system.

L-tryptophan is another amino acid,
or protein building block. The body first
converts it into 5HTP and then to
serotonin. Like certain other amino acids,
it is called 'essential' because the body
can't produce it. Although plentiful in
protein foods, cooking and processing
easily destroy it meaning deficiencies are
fairly common. Try Viridian L-Tryptophan
(£8.85 for 30 Vegicaps; available
nationwide).

MAGNESIUM

Along with contributing to a good night's
sleep, this mineral helps maintain normal
muscle and nerve function, keeps your
heart rhythm steady, supports a healthy
immune system and keeps bones strong.
Magnesium can also help regulate blood
sugar levels, and promote normal blood
pressure. Lack of the mineral inhibits
nerve cell communication, which leads
to cell excitability – something that can
contribute to stress and hamper a good's
night's sleep – while studies show that
good levels of magnesium can improve
sleep quality and reduce nocturnal
awakenings. BetterYou Magnesium Oil
Original Spray (£12.69 for 100ml, available
nationwide) delivers this essential mineral
directly into the skin tissue, efficiently
replacing magnesium faster than
traditional oral supplementation.

MELATONIN

The hormone melatonin regulates our
circadian rhythms – the cycle of activities
linked to our sleep-wake patterns. It's
produced naturally in the pineal gland after
the sun goes down, letting us know it's
time to fall asleep. Levels drop off
when we are exposed to light again in
the morning. Although melatonin hasn't
always been licensed for sale in the UK,
melatonin supplements have long been
used by those in the know to counter the
affects of jet lag. While many experts
believe occasional use is safe, there
is some concern that long-term
supplementation with synthesised
melatonin could, in fact, amplify insomnia.
This is because your body could
produce less melatonin as a result of
supplementation, which could interfere
with your natural sleep cycles. Still,
there is plenty of evidence that taking
a supplement such as Solgar Melatonin
10mg (£10.74 for 60, evitamins.com)
occasionally – when your sleep patterns
have gone awry due to a long-haul
flight, for example – can aid your sleep
in the short term.

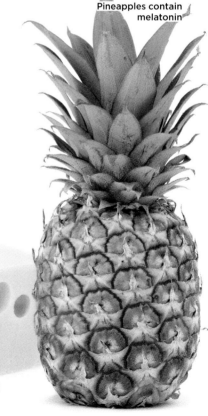

Pineapples contain
melatonin

Protein foods are a good
source of L-tryptophan

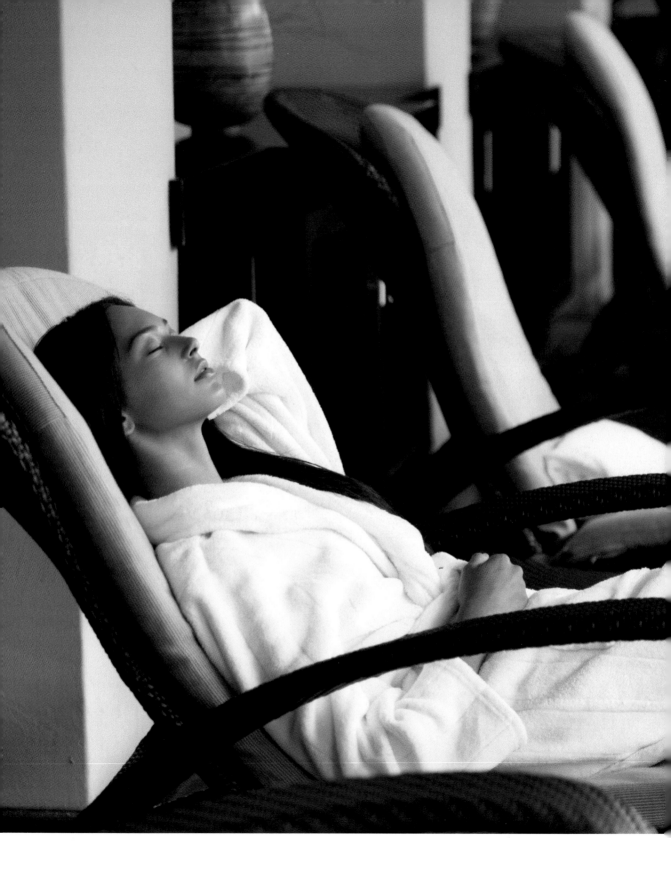

SOLVE YOUR
SLEEP PROBLEMS

For some people, hardcore insomnia's tough to shift. That's when you may need extra help. We have the low-down on how your GP can help you on p80, because sometimes you need short-term medical support to break a bad sleep pattern. Scientists are learning more all the time about the way your body clock affects your shuteye – work out how to tune into your own natural rhythms and harness them so you wake feeling restored (p94). And tap into the power of modern technology with our guide to the top sleep apps (p110). Fancy a more luxurious approach to a restful night? Turn to p120 for a round-up of the world's best sleep spas.

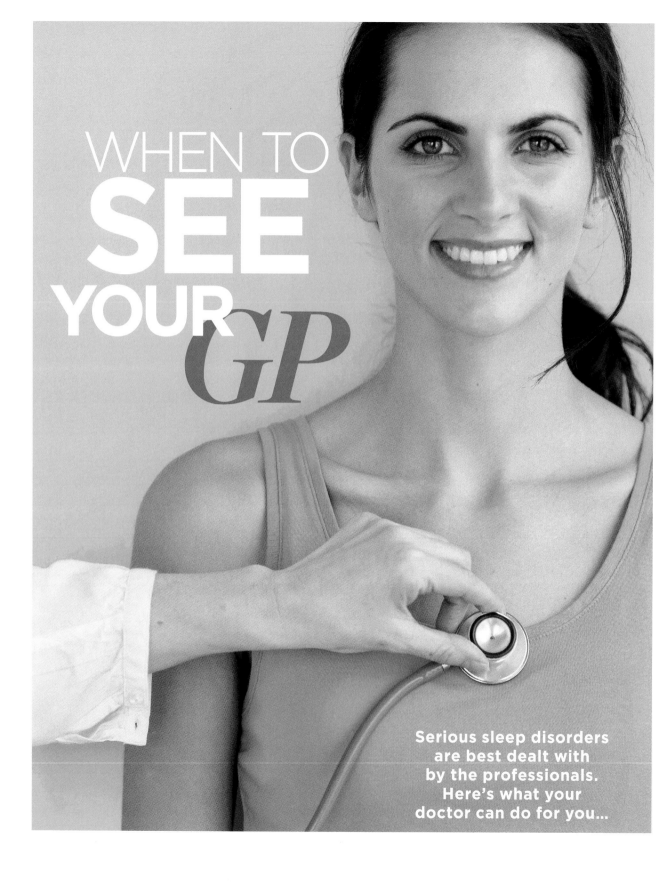

WHEN TO SEE YOUR *GP*

Serious sleep disorders are best dealt with by the professionals. Here's what your doctor can do for you...

While there's plenty you can do to help yourself get a good night's sleep, if nothing's working for you, it may be time to make an appointment to see your GP. This is especially true if lack of sleep is affecting your daily life and is turning into a long-term problem.

Your GP will probably ask you about your sleeping routine, your daily alcohol and caffeine consumption and your general lifestyle habits, such as diet and exercise, and can check your medical history for any illness or medication that may be contributing to your insomnia. Your doctor will also try to identify and treat any underlying health condition, such as anxiety, that may be causing your sleep problems.

Prescription sleeping tablets are usually only considered as a last resort and should be used for only a few days or weeks at a time as they are associated with side effects

As well as advising on things you can do at home that may help to improve your sleep (general sleep hygiene tips), your GP could recommend a special type of cognitive behavioural therapy (CBT) designed for people with insomnia (see Calm your mind, page 54). This is a type of talking therapy that aims to help you avoid the thoughts and behaviours affecting your sleep. It's usually the first treatment recommended, and can help lead to long-term improvement of your sleep.

Your GP may also refer you to a clinical psychologist. Prescription sleeping tablets, however, are usually only considered as a last resort and should be used for only a few days or weeks at a time. This is because they don't treat the cause of your insomnia and are associated with a number of side effects. They can also become less effective over time (see page 83 for more details).

Interrupted sleep is another reason to visit your GP. If you're waking up regularly

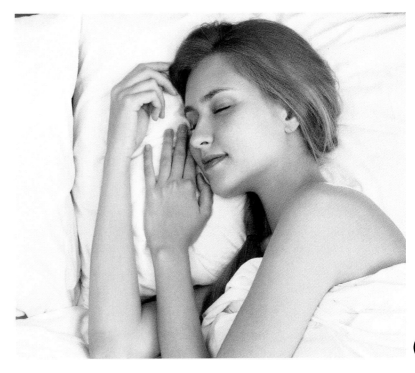

Lifestyle changes such as losing excess weight, cutting down on alcohol and sleeping on your side can reduce the symptoms of obstructive sleep apnoea

throughout the night, it could be a sign that you have obstructive sleep apnoea (see below), a common medical condition that's relatively easy to treat.

BEAT SLEEP APNOEA

Across the globe, around 100 million people are thought to have obstructive sleep apnoea (OSA), where the walls of the throat relax and narrow during sleep, interrupting normal breathing and disturbing your sleep.

During an episode, the lack of oxygen triggers your brain to pull you out of deep sleep – either to a lighter sleep or to wakefulness – so your airway reopens and you can breathe normally. These repeated sleep interruptions can make you feel very tired during the day. You'll usually have no memory of your interrupted breathing, so you may be unaware you have a problem – it's often a friend, family member or a partner who spots the signs of OSA, which include loud snoring, noisy and laboured breathing, as well as the well-known repeated short periods where not breathing is interrupted by sudden gasps or snorting.

Lifestyle changes such as losing excess weight, cutting down on alcohol and sleeping on your side can reduce the

DO YOU HAVE A SLEEP DISORDER?

A sleep disorder is broadly defined as a physical or psychological problem that impairs your ability to sleep or causes increased sleepiness during the day. Everyone can experience sleep problems from time to time. However, you might have a sleep disorder if you experience one or more of the following:

◆ Regularly experience difficulty sleeping
◆ Are often tired during the day, even if you slept for at least seven hours the night before
◆ Have a reduced or impaired ability to perform regular daytime activities
◆ Fall asleep while driving
◆ Struggle to stay awake when inactive, such as when watching TV or reading
◆ Have difficulty paying attention or concentrating at work, school or home
◆ Experience difficulties performing to your usual ability at work or school
◆ Often get told by others that you look tired
◆ Have difficulty with your memory
◆ Have slowed responses
◆ Have difficulty controlling your emotions
◆ Feel the need to take naps almost every day

symptoms. Your doctor could also recommend using a continuous positive airway pressure (CPAP) device, which prevents your airway closing while you sleep by delivering compressed air through a mask. Wearing a gum shield-like device to hold your jaw and tongue forward, increasing the space at the back of your throat while you sleep, can help, too.

Surgery may also be an option in rare cases, where OSA is thought to be the result of an unusual inner neck structure.

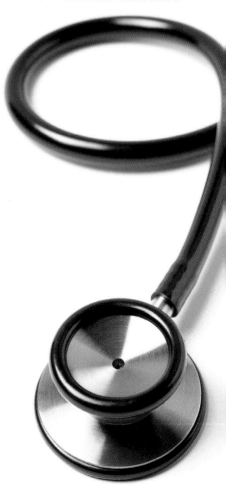

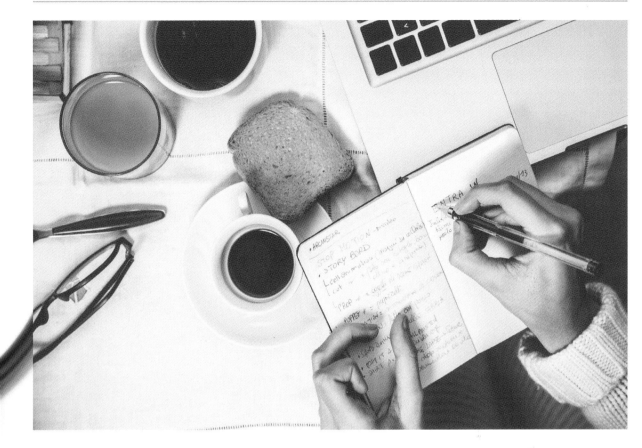

SLEEPING PILLS

Also known as hypnotic medicines, sleeping tablets encourage sleep. In the past, they were frequently used to help with insomnia, but they're prescribed much less often nowadays and generally will only be considered as a temporary measure to help ease short-term insomnia or if your insomnia is severe and hasn't responded to lifestyle changes or cognitive treatments.

Doctors are also usually reluctant to recommend sleeping tablets in the long-term because they just mask the symptoms without treating the underlying cause of insomnia. They can also result in potentially dangerous side effects, such as daytime drowsiness. Another concern is that some people become dependent on

Keep a sleep diary for at least a few days before you see your GP – this will help both you and your doctor get a better understanding of the roots of the problem

them. Sleeping pills can also stop working if you take them regularly.

If your doctor does recommend tablets – and you decide to take them – it's advisable to stick to the smallest effective dose possible for the shortest time (usually no more than two-to-four weeks) to minimise potential side effects.

KEEPING A SLEEP DIARY

If possible, keep a sleep diary for at least a few days before you see your GP – this will help both you and your doctor get a better understanding of the roots of the problem.

Each morning, make a note of things such as the time you went to bed and woke up, how long it took you to fall asleep, and the number of times you woke up during the night. Also, include if, and when, you take over-the-counter sleep aids, what you did in the hours before bedtime, what time you had your evening meal, whether you checked your phone or tablet in bed, what time you switched off the TV or if you exercised during the evening. In short, anything that could have an effect on your sleep patterns.

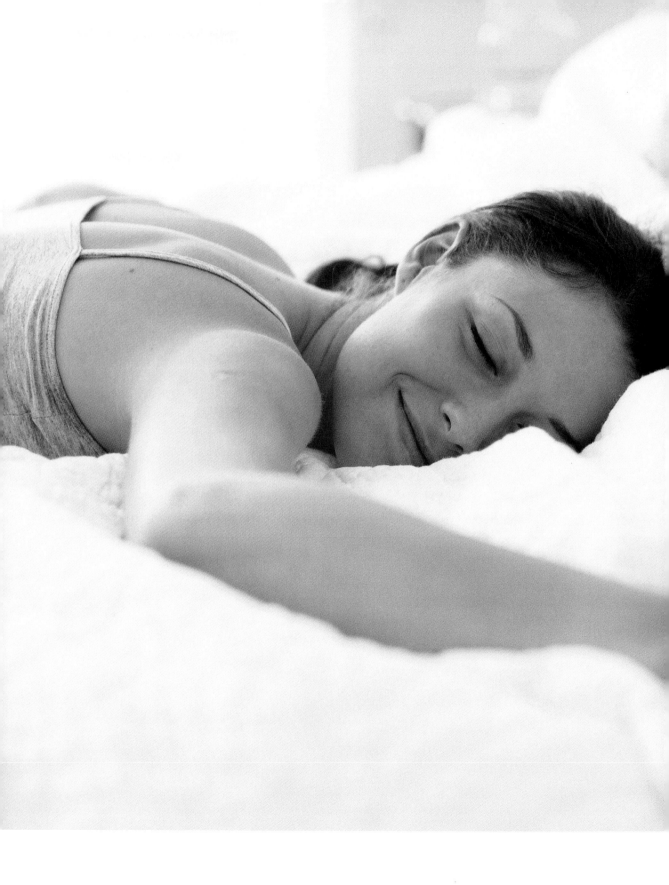

3

SURPRISING SLEEP DISRUPTORS

*I*t's not just stress and snoring that may be disturbing your slumber. Here are three common health conditions that might be keeping you awake at night – and how you can tackle them

1 NIGHT SWEATS

These aren't just associated with perimenopause – lots of women find they get night sweats pre-menstrually as well. It's all connected with dipping levels of oestrogen, either in the run-up to menopause, which can start to happen as early as your late thirties, or before your period. And hot flushes can wake you and make sleep uncomfortable.

WHAT CAN YOU DO?
'Dietary factors can aggravate hot flushes and night sweats, so avoid eating too late at night and cut back on fatty foods, sugar, caffeine and alcohol,' says nutritionist Emma Ross. You could also try the herb sage. Make a tea with fresh leaves. What you wear in bed counts as well – go for natural fibres such as cotton and silk, as artificial materials such as polyester will make sweating worse. Choose thin layers you can remove easily if you get too hot.

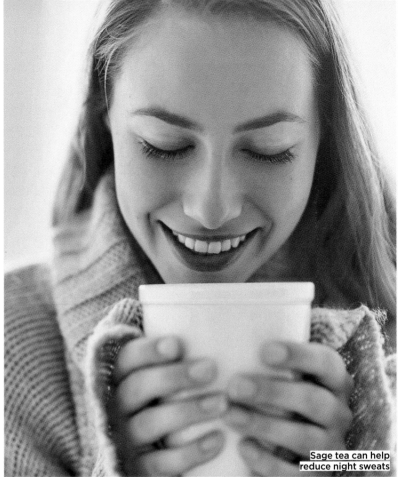

Sage tea can help reduce night sweats

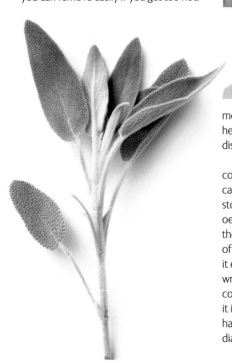

2 COUGHING

Obviously coughing occurs when you have a cold or flu – in which case it should pass with the virus. In the meantime, taking a decongestant can help you stay asleep without the cough disrupting your night.

If you constantly wake up coughing, it could be down to another, more chronic cause, such as acid reflux. This occurs when stomach acid escapes through the lower oesophageal sphincter and moves up into the oesophagus (food pipe). And reflux is often worse at night as lying down makes it easier for stomach acid to flow the wrong way. Asthma can cause nighttime coughing, too – and it's possible to develop it in adulthood, so don't assume you don't have asthma just because you weren't diagnosed as a child.

WHAT CAN YOU DO?
If you've recently starting waking with a cough, and there isn't an obvious reason for it, see your doctor. If they suspect asthma, they'll carry out tests and give you treatment – it's important to get diagnosed as untreated asthma could lead to a potentially life-threatening asthma attack.

'To help with acid reflux, avoid eating several hours before going to bed,' says Ross. This allows time for your latest meal to digest and move out of your stomach. You should steer clear of caffeine and alcohol in the few hours before bed, too, as these can cause the lower oesophageal sphincter to relax, making it harder for it to keep acid down. It's also a good idea to try elevating your head and chest in bed rather than lying flat – try putting some blocks under the top legs of your bed to tilt it up by about four inches.

Low levels of feelgood brain chemical dopamine may be connected to restless legs. And as dopamine falls at the end of the day, this may be why RLS tends to be worse at night

3 RESTLESS LEGS

Estimated to affect around three million in the UK, restless legs syndrome (RLS) causes a creepy-crawly discomfort in your legs, leading to the urge to jerk them about uncontrollably, particularly at night – so it can be very disruptive of sleep. It may not sound a serious condition, but some research has linked RLS with depression, and it can also indicate you may be at a higher risk of high blood pressure and a greater risk of type 2 diabetes. The latest research suggests there's a genetic link, and that low levels of feelgood brain chemical dopamine may be connected. As dopamine falls in everyone at the end of the day, this may be why RLS tends to be worse at night.

WHAT CAN YOU DO?

Don't hesitate to see your GP if you suspect you may be affected by RLS. Iron deficiency is sometimes an underlying cause, so see your doctor for a blood test to find out whether you need to take a prescription dose of iron to up your levels. A magnesium deficiency can also be linked, so you could try taking a supplement of this mineral. Keeping active during the day can help, and make sure you stay hydrated and follow a healthy diet with plenty of fresh fruit and veg.

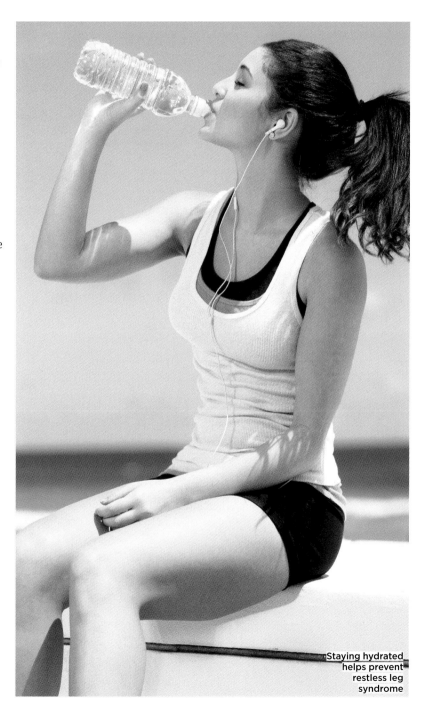

Staying hydrated helps prevent restless leg syndrome

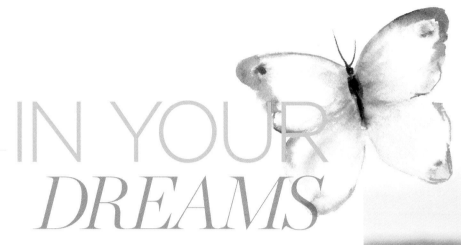

IN YOUR DREAMS

You probably dream each night, even if you don't know it. But what are dreams and can you choose the ones you want?

You're drinking coffee with Ryan Gosling, who's giving you some acting tips. Then a giant chicken strolls past and suddenly you're in front of a class, teaching geography. Yes, most dreams can seem nonsense – so what's the point of them? Strangely, experts still aren't sure. Some theories include emotional regulation – in other words, your mind is sorting through things that happened during the day – and memory consolidation, as your brain discards what's less important and banks the relevant stuff.

Think you rarely dream? According to independent sleep researcher Dr Neil Stanley, we all dream every night – it's just that you only tend to remember dreams if you wake up from one. You may not even realise you've woken – it might just be for a nanosecond – but it's enough to log the dream which makes it more likely that you will recall it the next day.

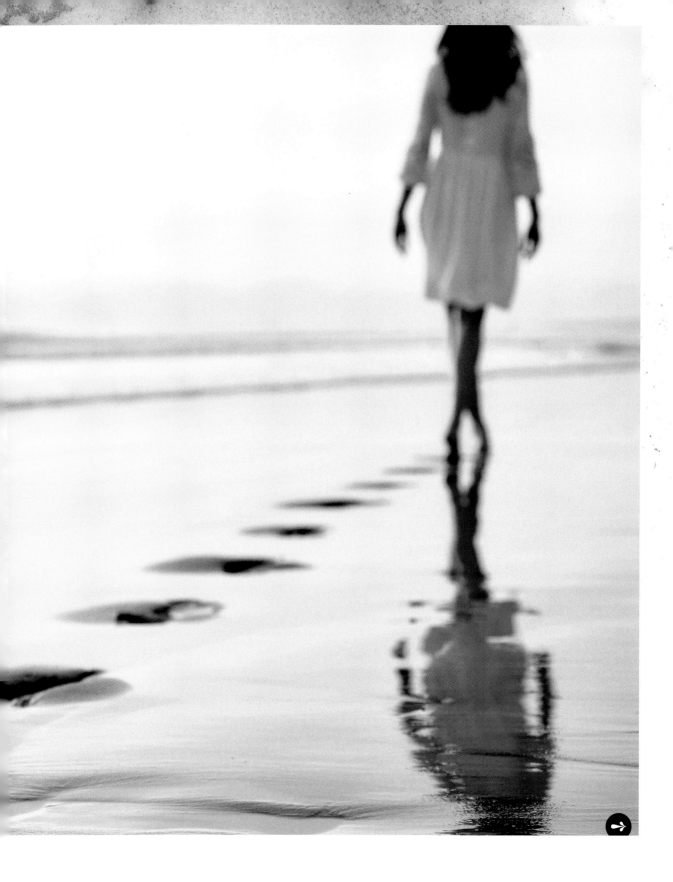

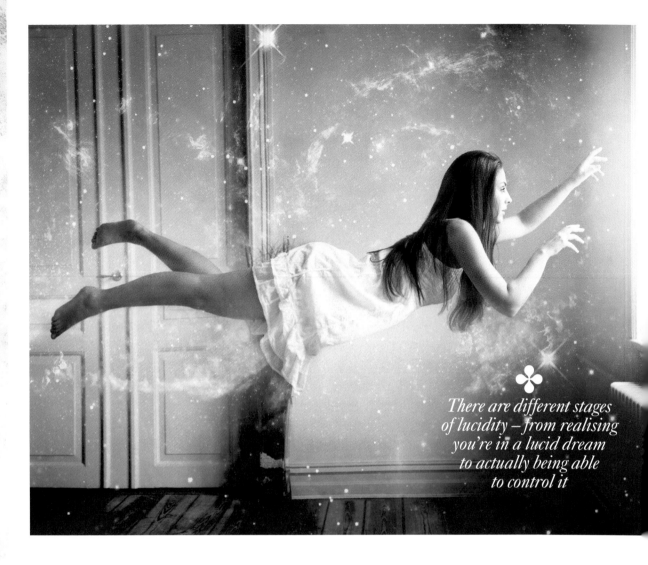

There are different stages of lucidity – from realising you're in a lucid dream to actually being able to control it

DO DREAMS GIVE YOU MESSAGES?

Some people swear they get important signs from their subconscious when they dream. A few common themes include:

✦ BEING CHASED According to dream interpreters, this usually means you're avoiding some important issues you don't want to face.

✦ FALLING This is said to mean you're feeling out of control or fearing failure. That's not necessarily a negative thing – it may just mean you need to relinquish your idea of a certain outcome.

✦ FLYING Most of us have had the uplifting experience of a dream in which we're soaring high in the sky. Usually, it's thought to mean that you are feeling free and unrestricted at this point in your life.

✦ BABIES Often, when there is a baby in your dream it is considered to represent your own inner self. How do you treat the baby? If it's neglected, it may be an indication that you need to be looking after yourself a bit better.

✦ TEETH Classically, teeth in dreams are thought to represent confidence and power. That's why losing your teeth is a common dream event – it may indicate you're feeling somehow fragile in life.

However, the jury's out on whether certain universal symbols or events in dreams mean the same thing for all of us. What's probably most important is how you feel in the dream – that might give a more accurate interpretation. For example, if you feel scared when you're falling, is some uncontrolled aspect of your life making you nervous?

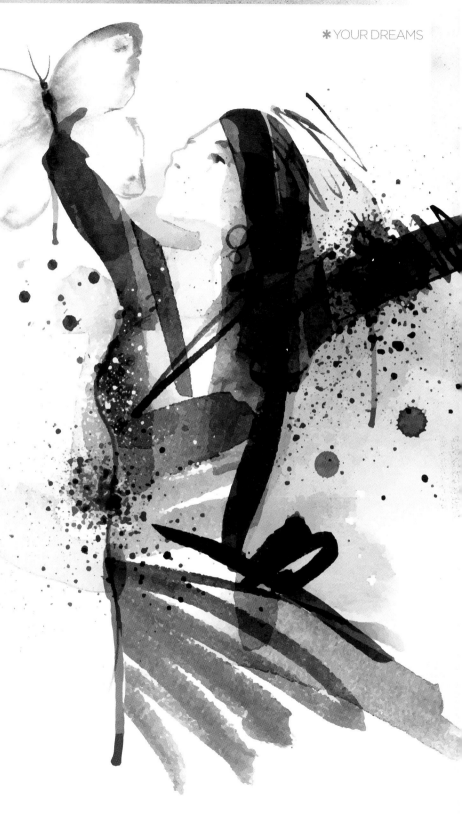

THE POWER OF LUCID DREAMING

'A lucid dream is one in which you become aware that you're dreaming,' says Dylan Tuccillo, co author of *A Field Guide To Lucid Dreaming* (Workman, $12.95). It's not just an intense dream – in a lucid dream, you know you're dreaming and can remember your daily life while you're in it. Research from Frankfurt University's Neurological Clinic and the Max Planck Institute of Psychiatry have found brain physiology actually changes once a dreamer becomes lucid, with greater activity in parts of the brain associated with self-assessment and self-perception – in other words, although you're asleep during a lucid dream, you're also aware.

There are different stages of lucidity – from realising you're in a lucid dream to actually being able to control it. And while being able to direct your own dream may sound enjoyable, experts believe there could be tangible benefits. 'By becoming consciously aware in dreams, you'll be able to tap into incredible amounts of knowledge and inspiration,' says Tuccillo. 'If you believe that the dream world is created by your subconscious mind, then it is the ideal location to let your creativity run wild.' (Paul McCartney apparently composed *Yesterday* after hearing it in a dream).

You could also solve problems – for example, rehearse a difficult conversation you need to have and see where your subconscious guides you with it. You might also get deep self-awareness and emotional healing, or work on addictions or phobias, as thinking and behaving a different way in a dream could help you lay down new neurological pathways.

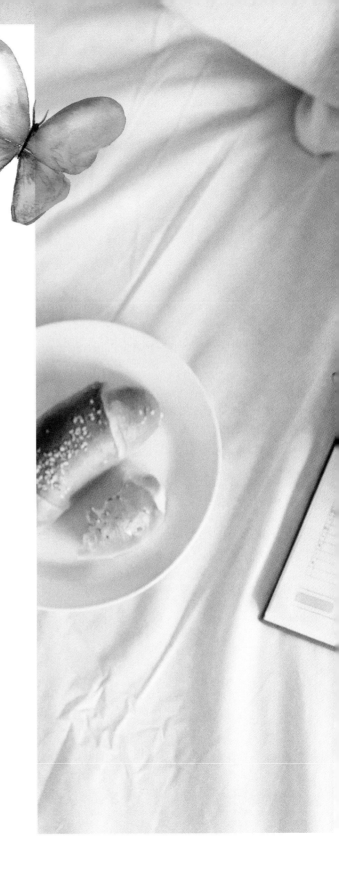

HOW TO LUCID DREAM

1 REMEMBER THEM

Start by becoming more conscious of the dreams you have. Simply setting the intention to recall them can help you do this. Keep a notepad by your bed, so as soon as you wake from a dream you can jot down the details. You'll soon notice you start becoming more conscious in your dreams.

2 SPOT RECURRING MOTIFS

'You'll notice you often dream about very similar things – for example, your sister, your pet, the ocean, anything,' says Tuccillo. 'These recurring elements are called dream signs and they're a powerful stepping stone to lucid dreams.' So go through your dream diary once you've kept it for a week or so, and start spotting recurring elements. Once you've found some dream signs, you can use them to step into a lucid dream – it's a little signaller. You can also use small gestures in your dream to check you're dreaming while aware – for example, look at your outstretched hand twice in quick succession without it changing in some way and you'll know that you are in a lucid dream state.

3 USE YOUR DREAMS

So you're in a lucid dream – what now? You could rehearse new mental habits, such as getting up early and running every other day, or being more assertive at work. Or you could ask what next step to take in your life – your subconscious often knows the answers to questions that puzzle you. Or just have fun – do something you enjoy and wake up the next morning feeling positive and inspired!

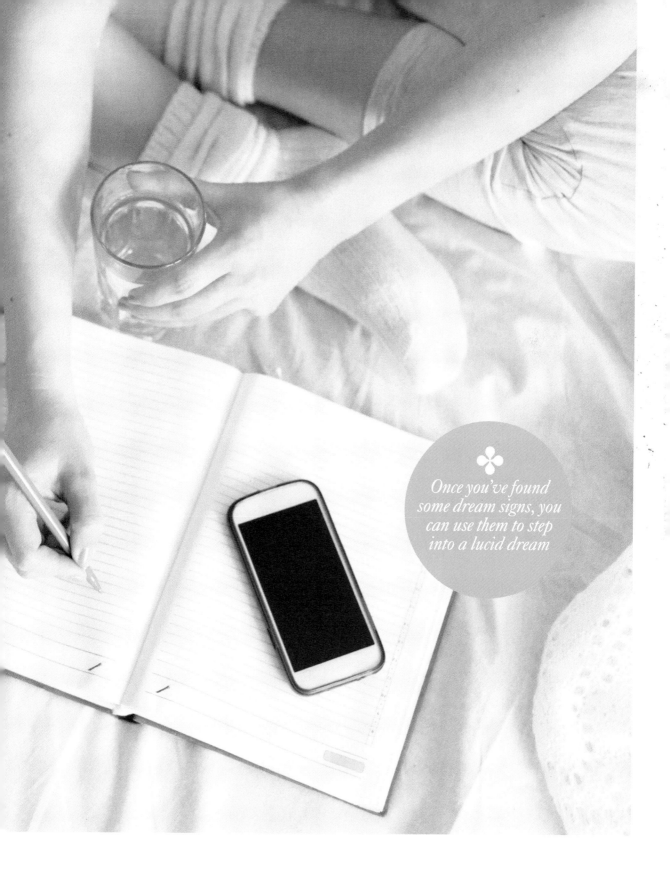

Once you've found some dream signs, you can use them to step into a lucid dream

BEAT THE
BODY
CLOCK
BLUES

YOUR INTERNAL BODY CLOCK HAS A MAJOR ROLE TO PLAY IN YOUR SLEEP QUALITY. BUT MODERN LIFE CAN INTERFERE WITH IT AND THROW SLEEP PATTERNS OUT OF KILTER. FIND OUT HOW TO GET YOURS TUNED UP AGAIN

DAY 13-14

Have you ever wondered why you feel sleepy at certain times of day? It's all to do with two systems in your body – sleep/wake homeostasis and your circadian biological clock. When you've been awake all day, sleep/wake homeostasis tells your body your need for sleep has accumulated and it's time to go to bed. It helps ensure you get enough sleep during the night to compensate for the time that you were awake during the day.

Most living things, including plants, animals and fungi, are governed by their circadian rhythms. They affect sleeping and eating patterns as well as core temperature and brain activity, and, in plants, determine the flowering period. Your circadian rhythm – often known as your body clock – regulates sleepiness and wakefulness. The rhythm dips and rises at different times of the day and night. It's a bit different for everyone – depending on whether you're naturally a lark or owl (see Owl or Lark, p24), but as a general rule, the strongest drive for sleep in adults is between 2am and 4am and also between 1pm and 3pm (hence the siesta), although you'll feel less sleepy in the daytime if you've had enough sleep at night. But

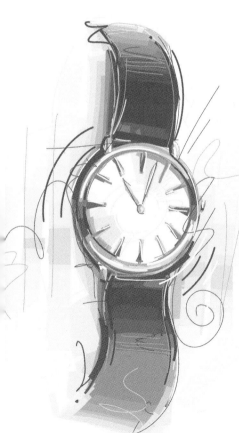

your body clock doesn't just make you feel tired. It also governs when you feel refreshed and alert – so it's why you can get up and about in the morning.

HOW DOES YOUR BODY CLOCK WORK?

Your body clock is controlled by a part of the brain called the suprachiasmatic nucleus (SCN), a group of around 20,000 cells in the hypothalamus, a section of your brain that responds to light and dark signals. Light travels from your eyes' optic nerves to the SCN, giving your internal clock the signal that it's time to be awake. The SCN sends signals to raise your body temperature and produce hormones such as cortisol, while suppressing the release of sleep-inducing hormone melatonin. When it's dark, on the other hand, the SCN triggers production of melatonin, which makes you feel drowsy – and it keeps churning it out during the night to keep you asleep. All life on earth is thought to be influenced by circadian rhythms – and scientists also know each individual cell in your body has its own body clock.

WHY MODERN LIFE CAUSES PROBLEMS

Before the invention of electricity, our ancestors would have had little choice but to stay in tune with the light and dark of day and night. They would have felt sleepy and gone to bed soon after sunset, and then woken with the sunrise – a pattern far removed from our modern lifestyles. From street lighting to television and computer screens, it's impossible to avoid the fact that the night is lit up. And let's face it, for most of us it would be impractical to go to bed at 7pm and wake at 4am. But there are ways to compromise and get a little closer to the sleep patterns we're designed to have – improving sleep quality and quantity. Turn the page to find how reset your body clock.

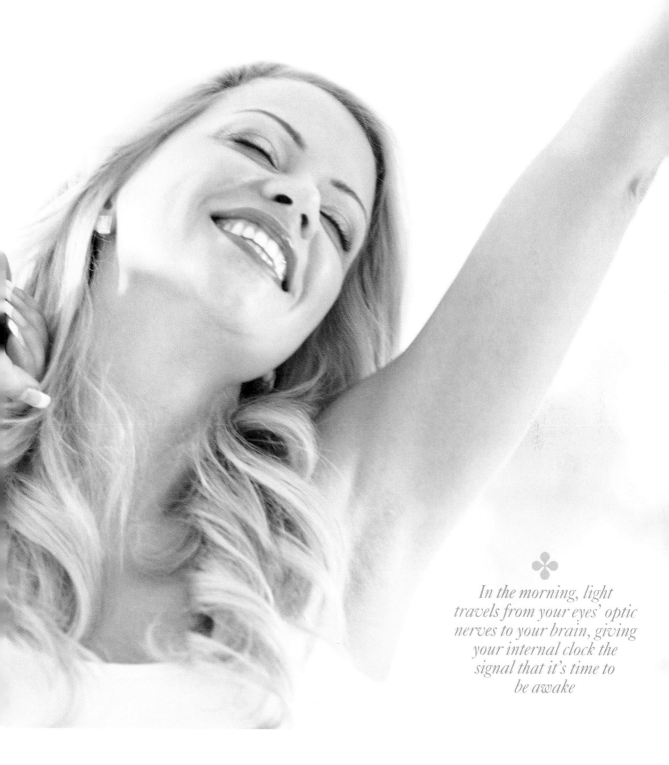

In the morning, light travels from your eyes' optic nerves to your brain, giving your internal clock the signal that it's time to be awake

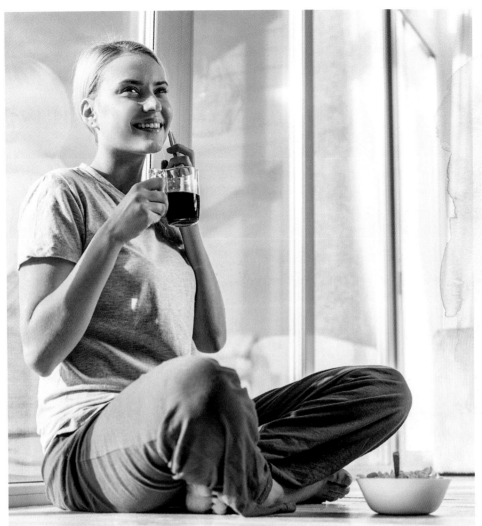

1. GET SOME EARLY MORNING SUN

This tells your body clock it's morning and time to be alert, effectively 'resetting' it each day. Even on a gloomy winter's morning, it's worth exposing yourself to some natural light so your body clock knows it's time to wake up – it will set the whole process in motion so you can sleep better at night. You could walk part of the way to work or even eat your breakfast by a window.

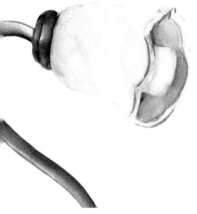

2. AVOID TOO MUCH NIGHT LIGHT

Russell Foster, professor of circadian neuroscience at Oxford University, points out that while we are not getting enough natural light during the day, we get too much artificial light at night. And that can throw your circadian rhythms out of whack. 'The circadian clock in the brain needs to be reset every day to 24 hours, and the 24-hour light-dark cycle performs this role,' explains Foster. 'The circadian pacemaker interprets light to mean daytime, even if it's actually night, and starts to readapt to the new "day-time" and shifts its timing.' Everything from shopping at all-night supermarkets to blue light from smartphones can contribute to evening wakefulness.

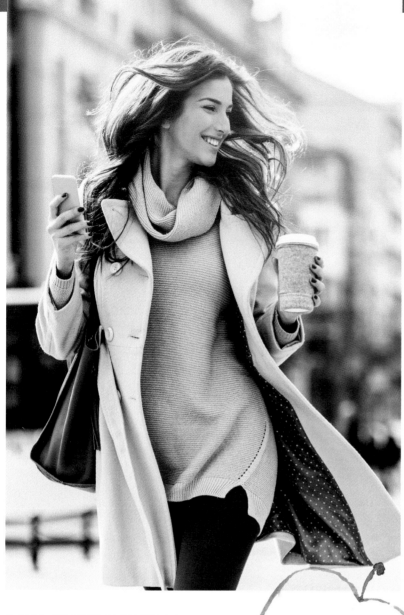

4. HEAD OUTSIDE FOR LUNCH

Being inside all the time rather than getting outdoors, may mean you're not getting enough sunlight to make vitamin D. And US research has found low levels of vitamin D may play a role in insomnia – scientists think that as there are vitamin D receptors in areas of the brain connected to the sleep-wake cycle, including the anterior and posterior hypothalamus, low vitamin D may contribute to missing out on sleep. Make sure you don't spend the whole day indoors – and when the weather's warmer, avoid using suncream all the time you're outside, as this stops your body synthesising vitamin D from sunlight. On average, on a warm spring or summer day, 15 to 20 minutes outside without suncream in the middle of the day is enough to generate sufficient vitamin D. But make sure you don't burn – very fair skins may need less time while darker skins may need more.

3. BE A CREATURE OF HABIT

Professor Foster recommends trying to go to bed and wake up at roughly the same times each day, so your body clock gets into a routine. But it's not even just about hitting the hay at regular times – eating at the same sorts of times each day could also help. And there may be other benefits – recent research from the University of Chicago, in the US, has suggested that snacking at irregular times of the day and night could throw your gut microbiome's rhythms out of whack – and this may be linked to weight gain. So keep to a routine when it comes to eating. The more you can stick to a daily routine, the better you're likely to sleep.

YOUR
INSOMNIA
TROUBLESHOOTER

Wide awake in the middle of the night? Here's what to do in those moments

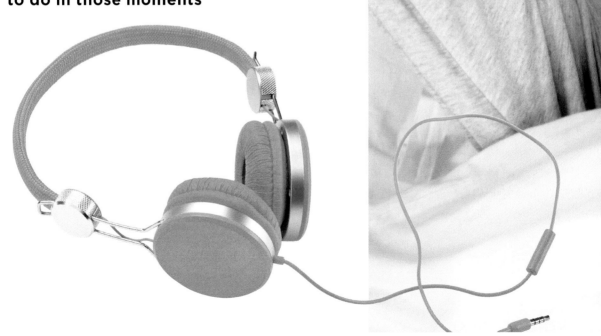

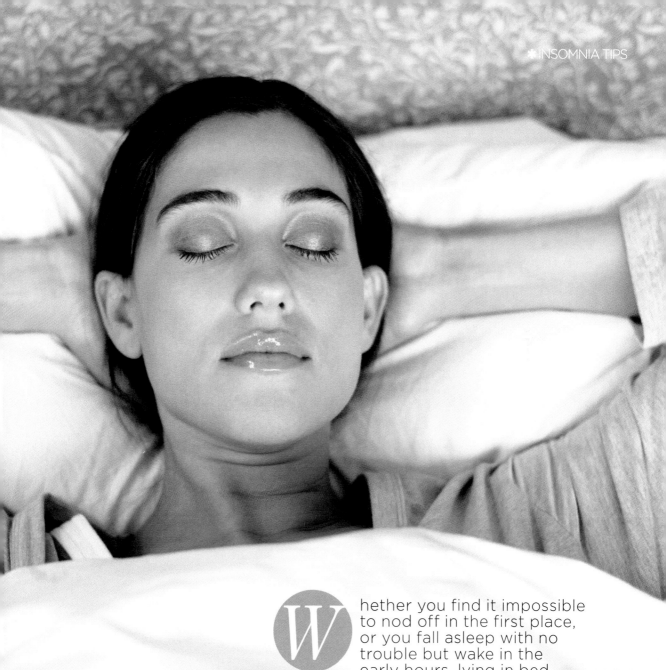

Whether you find it impossible to nod off in the first place, or you fall asleep with no trouble but wake in the early hours, lying in bed listening to the clock tick is a torment every insomniac will understand. In the long term, taking the steps outlined in the rest of this book is the best way to tackle sleep problems. But while you're putting those in place, what can you do to help yourself drift off again when you wake in the night? Try these expert tips.

1

WRITE OUT YOUR WORRIES

If you wake up at 2am panicking about work or DIY jobs you need to do, scribbling out your worries can be helpful. At times of stress, keep a notepad and pen by your bed so you can get those troublesome thoughts out of your head and onto paper. It might sound too simple to be effective, but if you keep the worries churning around in your mind, your brain will think there's a threat and keep you awake. The sooner you get the worries – or the things you need to remember – out of your head and onto paper, you'll relax, knowing you don't have to keep things at the front of your mind.

2

LISTEN TO SOMETHING SOOTHING

Focusing on something other than the voice in your head can distract you from worrying about lying awake, so you relax and fall asleep again. You could try a sleep hypnosis podcast or YouTube video, or something that isn't directly sleep-related, such as a relaxing radio play or story, or a lecture on something involving (just make sure it isn't anything too stimulating!) Or have a calming audiobook that's your fallback for those times you can't sleep. A classical music radio station can help you relax, too.

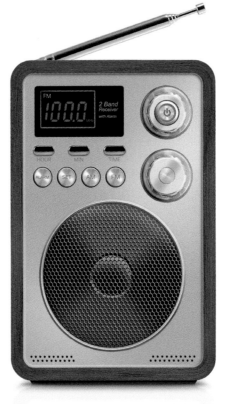

3

TRY NOT TO WORRY

Easier said than done, but it can be helpful to remind yourself waking in the night isn't as terrible as it seems. You've probably had more sleep than you realise and, it's worth remembering, while you're lying down, you're still resting, even if you're not asleep – so you're getting some of the benefits of bedtime. Thinking like this can help switch off your anxieties so your brain is relaxed enough to let you fall asleep again. It may be helpful to write out some of those reassuring thoughts during the day, so you can read them when you're lying awake in the night.

WHAT NOT TO DO

Don't keep checking the clock – you'll only panic yourself if you know how long you've been lying awake. In fact, if you're prone to waking in the night, keep the clock turned away from you.

Don't drink anything containing caffeine or sugar, such as hot chocolate, which may make you more wakeful.

Try not to talk to your partner – even if they're awake too – a conversation can be too stimulating, and you'll probably both get wound up about your inability to sleep.

Don't turn on a bright light – it will snap your brain straight into wide-awake mode. If you get up to read, try to use a light with a dim bulb, or turn a lamp around so that it isn't shining straight at you.

4 GET OUT OF BED

It may be the last thing you feel like doing, but according to independent sleep researcher Dr Neil Stanley, getting out of bed is often the best thing to do if you've been lying awake for more than around 15 minutes. Otherwise, you're likely to lie there feeling increasingly stressed, which means – of course – you'll find it even harder to nod off again. You need to break the association of your bed with being wakeful and tense. 'Go and get a drink of water from the kitchen, or sit in a chair in the living room and read for a bit,' he suggests. 'Only go back to bed when you start to feel sleepy.'

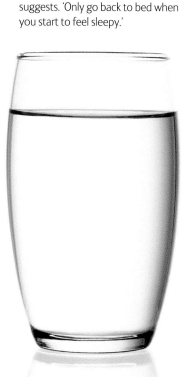

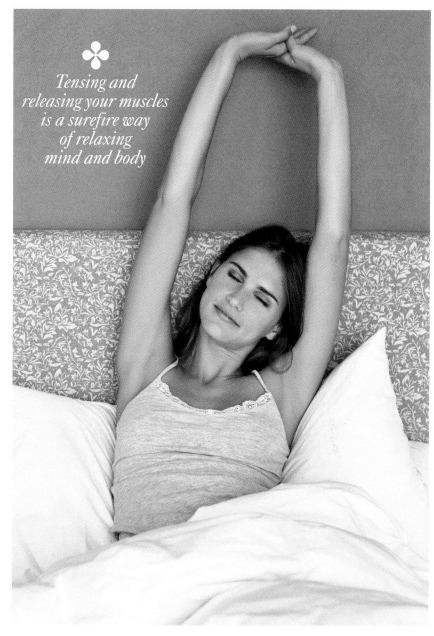

Tensing and releasing your muscles is a surefire way of relaxing mind and body

5 STRETCH IT OUT

Tensing and releasing your muscles is a surefire way of relaxing mind and body. Starting with your feet, tense your toes as tightly as you can, then release. Then grip the soles of your feet and relax. Continue moving up through your whole body doing this, until you get to your face. You may find you fall asleep long before you get to this point.

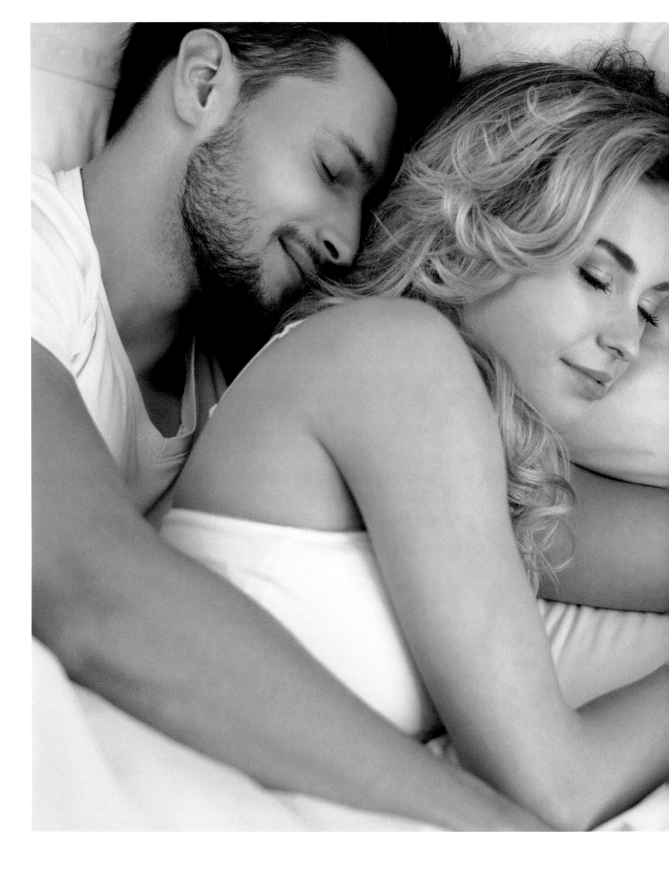

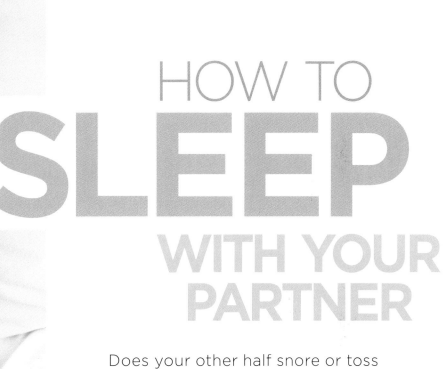

HOW TO
SLEEP
WITH YOUR
PARTNER

Does your other half snore or toss
and turn all night? Here's how to
ensure you both rest well

You think cuddling up with your partner should be something that happens easily and comfortably – but it's not unusual for sharing a bed to cause problems. In fact, one study found 29 per cent of people say their sleep is disrupted by their partner. Does that sound familiar? 'Ideally, couples should sleep separately,' says sleep researcher Dr Neil Stanley.

Although it's all too often seen as a sign your relationship is in trouble, in fact, the idea of couples needing to share a bed is a fairly recent one – our Victorian ancestors tended to sleep separately. And far from being bad for your relationship, Stanley points out that disturbed sleep causes a lot of stress and is, in fact, a major contributing factor to relationship breakdown – so going into separate rooms could preserve harmony at home.

Of course, not all couples are able to sleep separately – you may not have enough rooms in your home to do this. And you may simply be reluctant to sleep apart from your beloved. So here are ways to solve some of the most common problems of sharing a bed with your significant other...

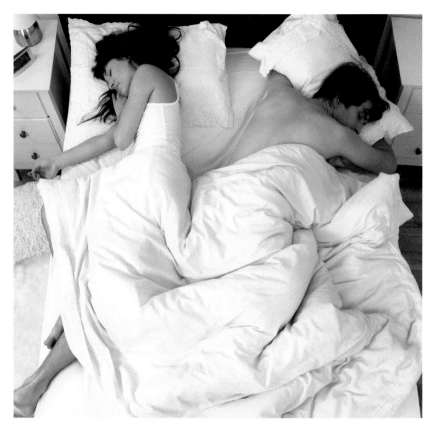

THE ISSUE:
THEY'RE RESTLESS

Some people move around in bed a lot more than others. But that can be really disturbing to the person they share with. Make sure your restless partner avoids too much sugar and caffeine during the day – both of these can cause a disturbed night's sleep with lots of tossing and turning. But choosing the right bed can be the most sensible answer. Look into getting a double bed that zips down the middle, so, while you're still sharing the bed, you effectively have different mattresses. That will reduce some of the movement disturbance you're experiencing. A memory foam mattress will transfer less motion across the bed, too.

THE ISSUE:
LARK VS OWL

When one of you is a lark but the other's a night owl, that can cause problems. It's particularly difficult for the person who goes to bed late and hopes to sleep later to make up for it, says Stanley. 'You are in a lighter sleep in the hours just before you wake up, so you'll be woken up more easily at this time,' he says. The person who goes to bed earlier, meanwhile, is more likely to be in a deep sleep by the time their partner hits the sack, so less likely to be woken. If you can't compromise on bedtime, try to protect yourself from being disturbed – Stanley recommends earplugs and an eyemask.

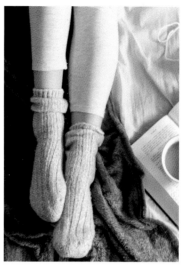

THE ISSUE:
TEMPERATURE CONTROL

So you're always cold in bed and your partner's usually too hot? Stanley recommends investing in two separate single duvets instead of sharing one larger one. That way, you can each choose the thickness that works for you. Or you could go for multiple separate blankets so you can each adjust the temperature on your side of the bed. These measures also solve the problem of duvet-thieving...

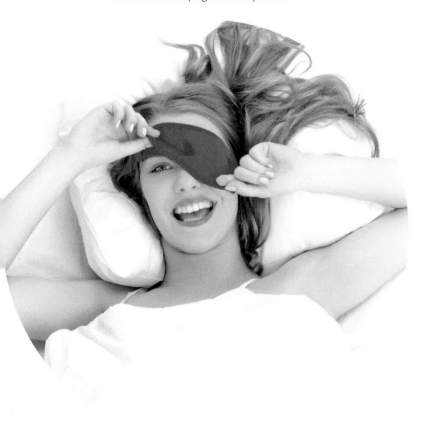

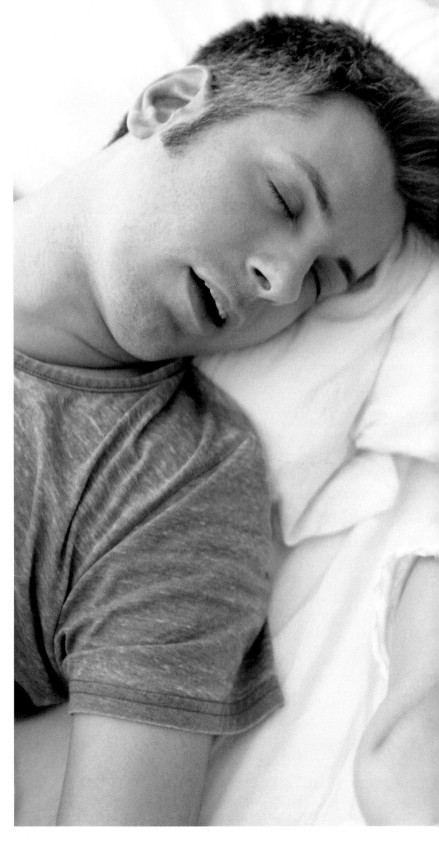

THE ISSUE:
THEY SNORE

This is a common cause of trouble and one that can be difficult to resolve. The first step is to encourage your partner to get help for themselves. That's particularly important if they snore very loudly as this can be a sign of sleep apnoea (see p82), a potentially dangerous condition that causes people to temporarily stop breathing in their sleep and can be linked to heart disease and other conditions. Suggesting your partner avoids alcohol and sedating antihistamines can also help lower the chances they'll snore, as can encouraging them to sleep on their side rather than their back. Meanwhile, for you, earplugs can help cut some of the noise – but go for some especially designed for the partners of snorers. You can find earplugs that cut down some of the volume of snoring at britishsnoring.co.uk

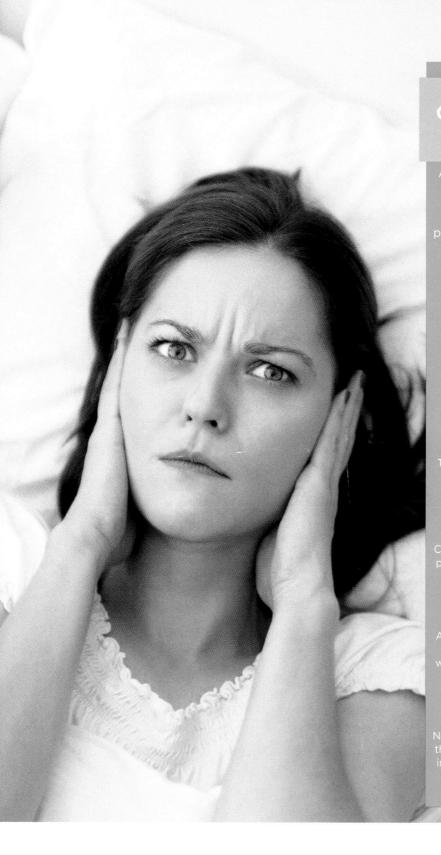

WHAT YOUR COUPLE SLEEPING POSITION SAYS ABOUT YOU

According to a psychological study for bed company Dreams, the way you curl up – or not – in bed with your partner can tell you a lot about your relationship. Here are some of the most common positions and what they may mean...

Sleeping back to back and far apart

While it may not look the most intimate, this is one of the most common sleeping positions for couples, and suggests you feel secure and relaxed with each other.

Spooning

This usually indicates the partner cuddling from behind feels protective of the other.

Back to back and touching

Common in new relationships, this position shows both partners feel relaxed with each other.

With your head on their chest

A very intimate sleeping position, this suggests you feel romantic with each other – you may be in a relatively new relationship.

One partner takes up most of the bed

Not surprisingly, this indicates that this partner tends to be dominant in the relationship and may make most of the big decisions.

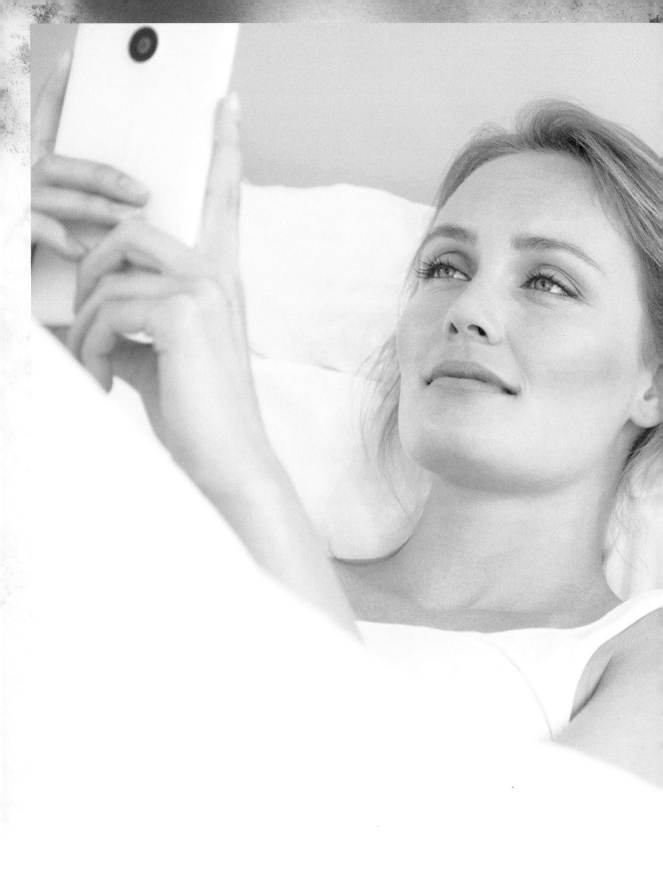

THERE'S AN
APP
FOR THAT...

O K, all the experts agree the bedroom is no place for your smartphone. And yes, browsing through Tinder before you turn out the light is a definite no-no. But there's one exception to the phone-in-bed rule: listening (or tracking) can help you sleep. Here's our pick of the apps that might help you get more shuteye.

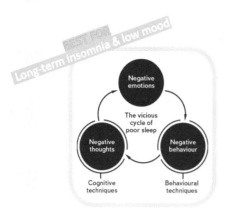

MORE THAN JUST A SLEEP APP

Sleepio is a six-week online sleep programme that's been clinically proven to help people with long-term sleep problems. It's based on cognitive behavioural therapy (CBT) techniques and was designed by a team of leading sleep experts and psychologists, including Professor Colin Espie from the University of Oxford. And it's tailored to each user.

In 2015, the app was independently tested by an NHS service and found not only to alleviate sleep problems, but also to relieve depression and anxiety in 65 per cent of users. It's now offered as an intervention on the NHS in some areas. Users take a test to identify their personalised Sleep Score, then learn proven sleep improvement techniques from 'The Prof', an animated sleep expert. It also syncs with popular activity and sleep trackers (such as Fitbit and Jawbone) to turn their data into something useful. In a survey, users saw a 58 per cent increase in daytime energy and concentration, and 62 per cent fewer awakenings during the night.

Sleepio, from £3.84 a week, sleepio.com

THE BUDDHA WITHIN

The Buddhify meditation app has been the number one app for health and fitness in more than 40 countries. Since its launch, people have used it to learn how to be more mindful and have meditated with it for a total of 14 million minutes! Last year, the iOS version of the app was relaunched with double the content, so it's worth another look if you've tried it in the past. There are now more than 80 meditation tracks lasting over 11 hours, covering all sorts of situations from commuting to stress at home. So it's helpful for easing anxiety or getting some quiet time during the day, as well as by night. Notably, some of the most popular tracks are the sleep meditations. There are six tracks called 'Going to sleep', ranging from five to 12 minutes long, all designed to help you nod off more easily. Then there are six more called 'Can't sleep', which help quieten down an active mind if you're wakeful during the night. Users like the fact most of the meditations are short, so they're easy to fit into a busy day.

Buddhify costs £1.99 for android, Buddhify2 is £3.99 for iOS

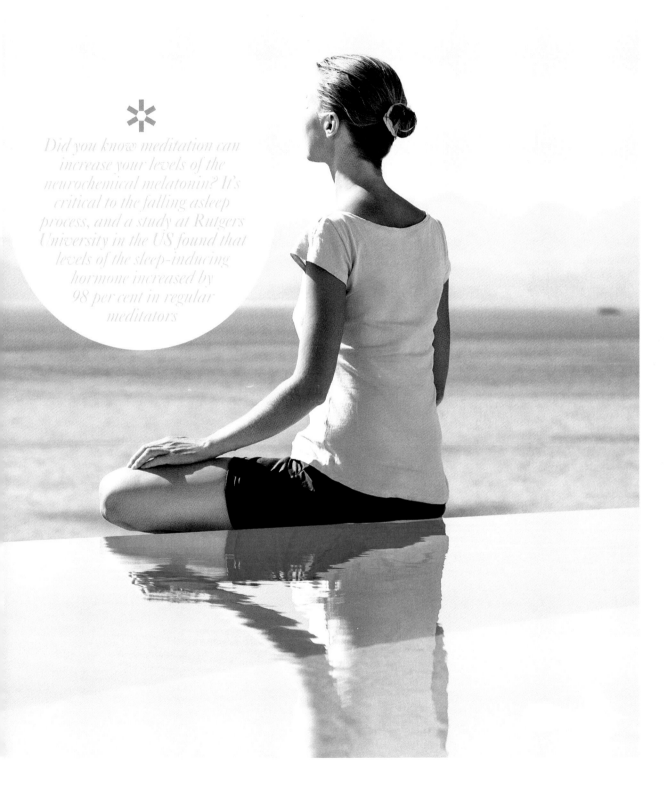

✳

Did you know meditation can increase your levels of the neurochemical melatonin? It's critical to the falling asleep process, and a study at Rutgers University in the US found that levels of the sleep-inducing hormone increased by 98 per cent in regular meditators

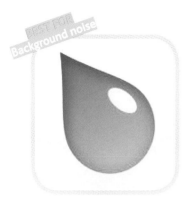

LET IT RAIN

Perhaps you like to fall asleep to white noise or soothing sounds from nature. Or maybe you're staying away from home and need to drown out distracting noise such as the hotel air conditioning, snoring from the room next door or a ticking clock. Rain Rain is a super simple but popular app that has 25 sounds from nature to lull you to sleep. As the name suggests, there are lots of variations on rain (Thunderstorm, City Rain, Rain on a Tent), but also other comforting sounds such as a crackling fire or ocean waves. You can mix sounds as well, and set a timer so they gradually fade out when you choose.
Rain Rain app, free, iTunes and Google Play

Ever wondered why calming sounds lull you to sleep? Because the brain perceives them as non-threatening enough to block out more threatening sounds, says a US study

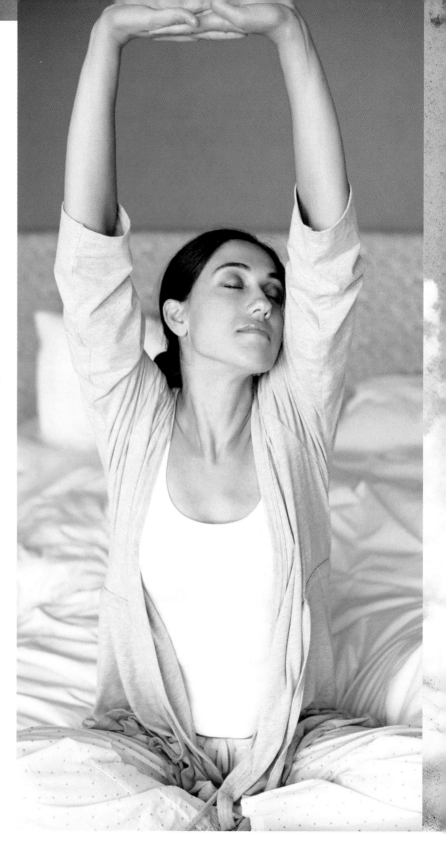

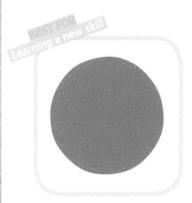

JOIN THE HEADSPACE TRIBE

You've probably heard of Headspace – the meditation app that's a personal trainer for the mind – even if you've not yet downloaded it. This app is a huge success story that's helped make meditation easy and understandable for the masses. What started as a simple way for people to get some daily 'time out', developed by a former Buddhist monk, has become a worldwide phenomenon worth more than £25 million. It currently has in excess of five million users.

If you've ever felt intimidated by how to meditate, simply sign up and follow the 10-minute guided sessions, narrated by Headspace founder Andy Puddicombe. You'll soon get the idea. If you like it, you can upgrade to the more bespoke version. There are exercises of different lengths, designed for sleep, anxiety, focus and many more needs. And if you want to make a commitment to learning to meditate, you can buddy up with other users to motivate each other.

Basic Headspace app, free; upgrade from £3.74 a month, headspace.com

BEDTIME STORIES FOR GROWN UPS

If ambient noises and breathing exercises aren't your thing, how about being read a story as you go to sleep? Sleep Stories is new feature on the meditation app Calm.com. It consists of 23 short stories, narrated by some familiar names. Described as 'tranquilising tales', they range from classic children's stories (such as *The Velveteen Rabbit*), to non-fiction nature essays; extracts from Shakespeare to some original stories created by mindfulness experts. They even have Ben Stein, the actor who played the boring economics teacher in 80s film *Ferris Bueller's Day Off*, reading from Adam Smith's economics text, *The Wealth of Nations* – for those who find complex ideas and monotonous voices soporific...

'Remember when you were young how much you enjoyed listening to a bedtime story,' says Alex Tew, co-founder of Calm. 'It was comforting, relaxing and soothing. Sleep Stories are the adult equivalent. When you're a child, you have much less on your mind and sleep comes easily. Sleep Stories are meant to take you back to a simpler mental state and let your brain relax and prepare for a deep rest, just as it did when you were young.'

Sleep Stories are available via the Calm app, which costs £9.99 a month (there's a seven-day free trial). Visit calm.com

A KINDER ALARM

Sleep Cycle Alarm Clock is a nifty app that promises to wake you gently in the mornings, rather than shocking you out of deep sleep. How does it work? You put your phone on your bedside table (or in your bed, for some phones). While you snore away it uses sound analysis to track your movements and map your sleep cycles: light, deep and REM. Then an alarm clock wakes you during your lightest cycle, which makes you feel as if you've woken naturally without using an alarm clock. It works by using a wake-up phase that ends at your desired alarm time, and you can go about your day feeling better rested. We know, it sounds unbelievable, but the app was crowned one of the most innovative in the Best of App Store 2016 round-up and has received some great reviews. Fans swear it's changed their morning mood. You can also use the app to look at your sleep cycles every night, to monitor how well you're sleeping overall.

Sleep Cycle Alarm Clock, from £1.99, sleepcycle.com

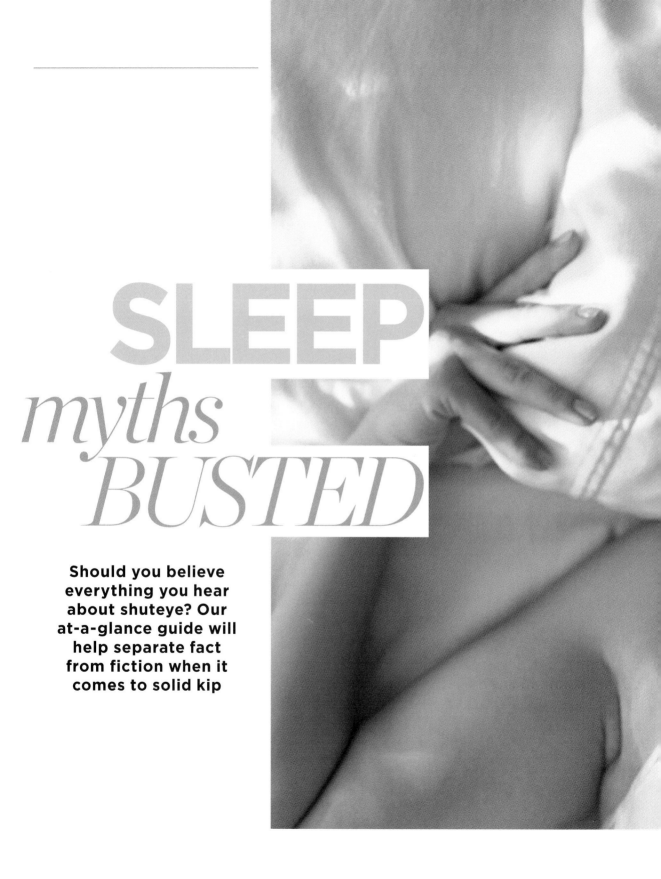

SLEEP
myths
BUSTED

**Should you believe
everything you hear
about shuteye? Our
at-a-glance guide will
help separate fact
from fiction when it
comes to solid kip**

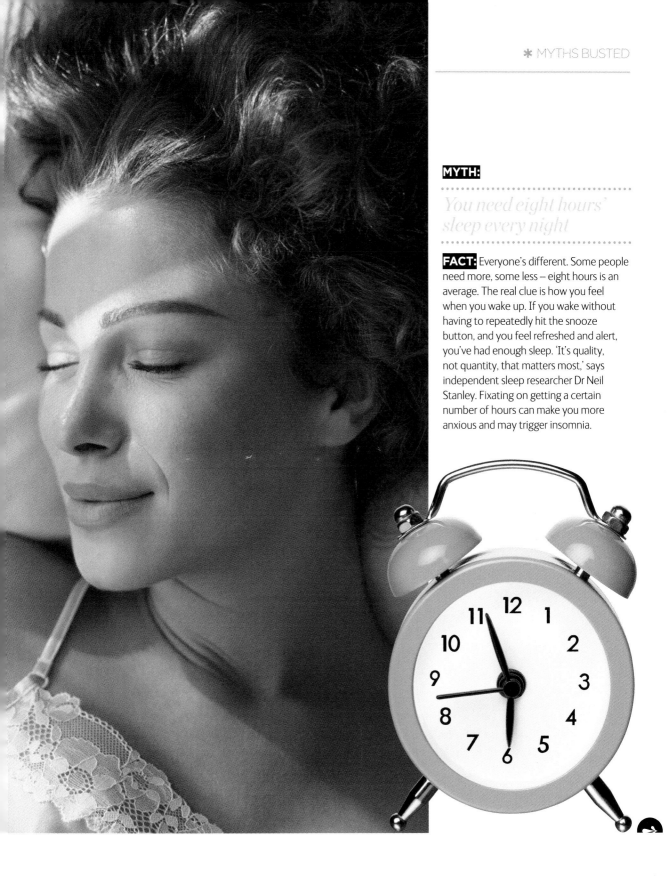

MYTH:

*You need eight hours'
sleep every night*

FACT: Everyone's different. Some people need more, some less – eight hours is an average. The real clue is how you feel when you wake up. If you wake without having to repeatedly hit the snooze button, and you feel refreshed and alert, you've had enough sleep. 'It's quality, not quantity, that matters most,' says independent sleep researcher Dr Neil Stanley. Fixating on getting a certain number of hours can make you more anxious and may trigger insomnia.

MYTH:

Caffeine too close to bed affects your sleep

FACT: It's true that caffeine can cause wakefulness. But it depends on your sensitivity to it. 'Doing something you enjoy, which relaxes you, is most important for helping you sleep,' says Stanley. And for those who aren't particularly sensitive to caffeine, having a coffee in the hours before bed may do more good than harm. But if you've noticed a link between caffeine and a poor night's sleep, avoid it from the afternoon onwards – and that includes coffee, tea, chocolate and painkillers, as some contain caffeine.

MYTH:

You can make up for sleep you lose

FACT: Having late nights at the weekend and then trying to compensate during the week can lead to a phenomenon known as 'social jet lag', where your bodyclock gets confused by irregular bedtimes. The occasional late night won't hurt, but if you do it regularly you won't be able to make up for it.

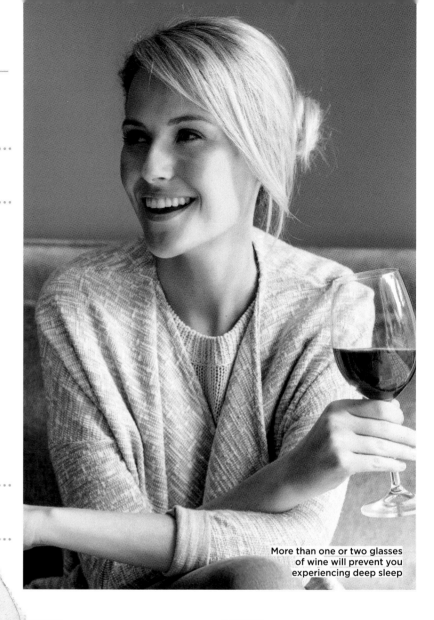

More than one or two glasses of wine will prevent you experiencing deep sleep

MYTH:

Wine helps you sleep better

FACT: A glass or two may help you nod off. But overdo it and your sleep will be disrupted. Excess alcohol affects the deeper stages of sleep, which is one of the reasons you feel so tired when you have a hangover, even if you feel you've spent a longer time in bed.

MYTH:

Sleep restores you physically

FACT: Strange as it may sound, experts don't fully understand the purpose of sleep. The thinking is it may be more about mental than physical restoration. So sleep is even more important to us than our ancestors, as we're more likely to have jobs that rely on brain power than physical work.

MYTH:

The more sleep you have, the better

FACT: Harvard research found sleeping for nine hours or more on a regular basis can actually be detrimental for your health, raising the risk of poor quality sleep. If you enjoy the odd lie-in, don't worry. But frequently sleeping for more than nine hours might cause wellbeing problems.

MYTH:

Afternoon naps are good for you

FACT: Up to a point. Research from Spain found a brief nap helps heart health, reduces stress and improves alertness and memory. But try to limit your nap to less than half an hour – fall asleep for longer and you'll go into a deeper phase of sleep, which might interfere with your kip at night. Twenty minutes is perfect for power naps – and a quick kip really does have benefits. A 2008 study in Dusseldorf found simply the process of falling asleep triggers active memory processes. And while it may sound counterintuitive, it's a good idea to have a coffee before your siesta – caffeine takes up to 30 minutes to kick in so having it before you doze off means you'll wake more alert. Clever!

MYTH:

An evening workout will affect your sleep

FACT: Vigorous exercise too late in the day is sometimes associated with poor

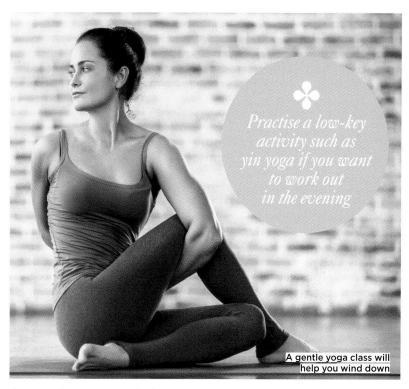

Practise a low-key activity such as yin yoga if you want to work out in the evening

A gentle yoga class will help you wind down

sleep at night – it raises your body temperature and triggers the release of adrenaline, both of which can cause wakefulness. But if you have no other time to work out, it's much better to be active in the evening than not at all. Lack of exercise is far more likely to keep you awake. That said, it might be preferable to practise more low-key activity if you have to work out in the evening – wind down with a gentle jog or a yin yoga class.

MYTH:

Having your pet in your bedroom is relaxing

FACT: Lots of us let our cats or dogs sleep in our bedrooms – or even on or in bed with us. You may find it comforting but most surveys show having Fido in bed is likely to be disruptive. Think pouncing on your toes, moving under the covers and whining for food in the early hours.

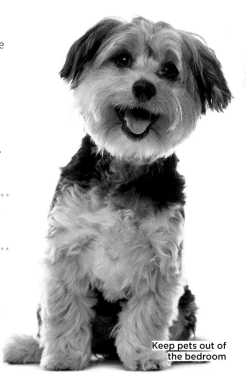

Keep pets out of the bedroom

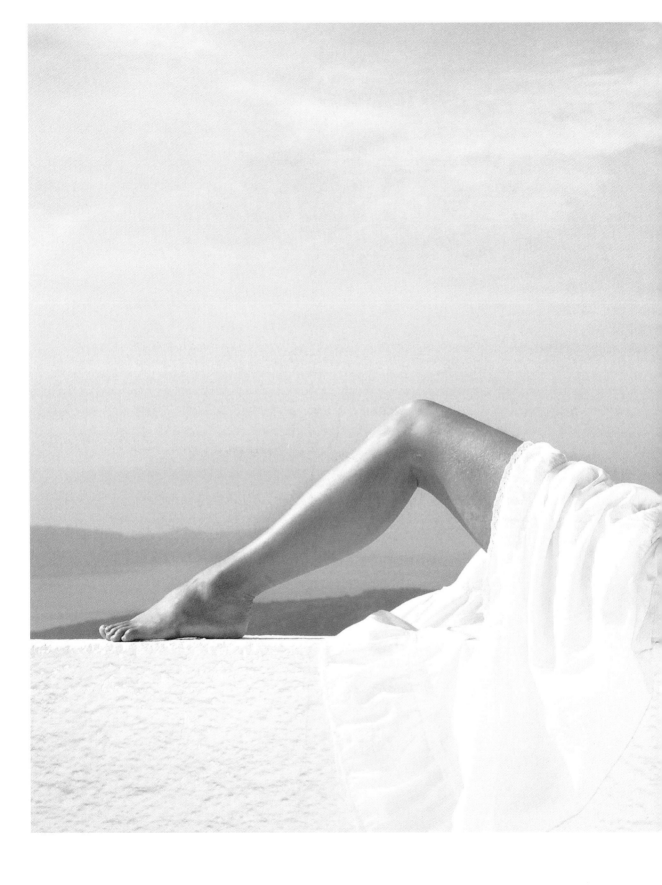

RETREAT TO
SLEEP

**From luxurious relaxation breaks
to slumber-inducing day-spa
packages, we've rounded up
the best sleepy getaways
and workshops...**

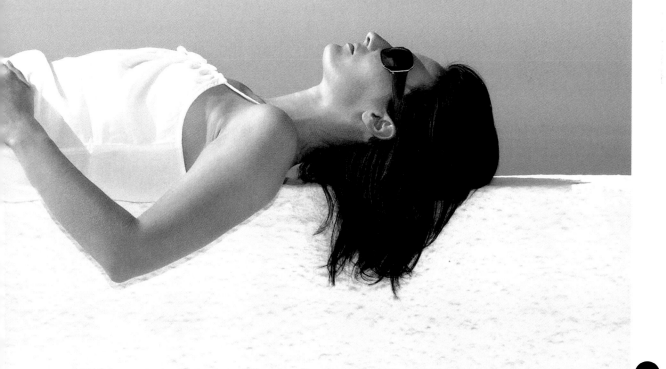

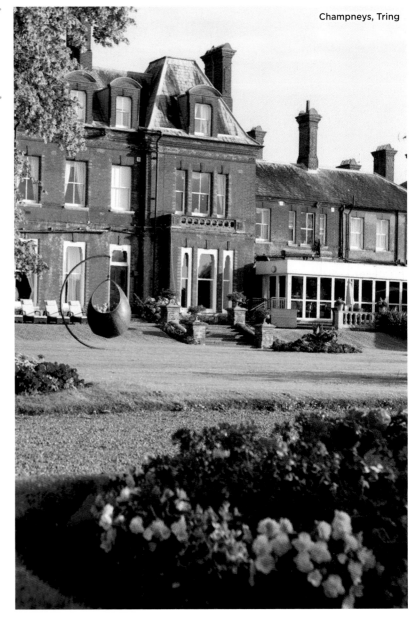

Serious sleep courses

Struggling with stubborn sleep issues? These retreats will help you get to grips with your insomnia.

● SLEEP RETREAT, CHAMPNEYS TRING

Check in to the famous health spa for a Sleep Retreat led by one of the world's top sleep experts, Professor Jason Ellis. Treat yourself to a relaxing combo of super-soothing massages and dips in the thalassotherapy pool, along with sessions to help you understand the reasons behind your sleep problems, and discover techniques for dealing with them. Tailored to you, the two-night break is designed to leave you feeling thoroughly blissed out – and you'll also leave with lots of takeaway tips on getting good sleep.

Cost: From £499 for two nights, including all meals, fitness classes and spa.

Find out more: champneys.com

● THE SLEEP RETREAT, HAMPSHIRE

Developed by a former insomniac after his own sleep issues were successfully treated, your stay is based around four pillars of sleep: the clinical side, involving CBT to tackle unhelpful beliefs; nutrition; wellness activities, including yoga, walking and massage; and social activities such as art and music. Think luxury rather than boot camp – you're here for an über-indulgent week where you will focus on yourself and learn lifelong skills.

Cost: Bespoke sleep weeks cost around £3,600.

Find out more: the-sleep-retreat.com

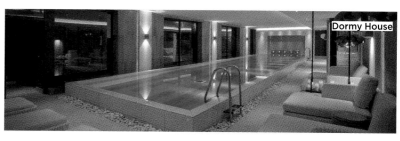
Dormy House

Get away for a day

You don't have to stay at a retreat to get the sleep spa benefits – these one-day packages will all give you some serious shuteye too...

● THE SLEEP SCHOOL, LONDON

Don't have the time or cash to make it to a proper spa or retreat? The Sleep School's one-day workshops, devised by expert Dr Guy Meadows, give you all the essential tools you need for proper shuteye. In a group, you'll learn practical tips for quality sleep. It may not be indulgent but it works, according to Dr Meadows' impressive testimonials.
Cost: From £149
Find out more: thesleepschool.org

● ESPA LIFE AT CORINTHIA, LONDON

Enjoy the one-day Mindful Sleep package at one of London's leading luxury hotels. It targets physical and mental tension, with a relaxing body massage using hot stones and warm oil, a super-soothing scalp massage, and guided mindful breathing techniques and visualisations you can take away to lull you to sleep at home. You'll get the chance to have a two-hour yogic nap and then indulge in a delicious meal from the spa's Mindful Food Menu.
Cost: £280
Find out more:
espalifeatcorinthia.com

Yogic sleep is a powerful relaxation technique. When practised successfully, it can be as restorative as sleep – except that you remain fully aware throughout

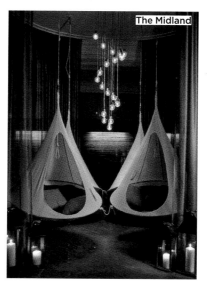
The Midland

● TOP TO TOE SPA DAY, DORMY HOUSE, COTSWOLDS

A day of indulgence designed to help you relax deeply and shake off stress. It gives you exactly what it says on the tin – a full programme of treatments from your head to your feet, including a tension-busting scalp massage, a delicious foot scrub, and a full body scrub and massage. You'll get a light meal and a Temple Spa Silent Night Kit to take away.
Cost: £195
Find out more: dormyhouse.co.uk

● SERENE SLEEP DAY AT THE SPA AT THE MIDLAND, MANCHESTER

This exclusive ESPA package will leave you seriously blissed out, and promises to put you back on the path to restorative slumber if you've been going through a stressful time. You'll enjoy a hot stone back massage, working on energy points to clear blockages and detoxify you, and a facial massage with rose quartz crystals to target the tension you hold in your facial muscles. The treatment is finished off with a deep scalp massage to blitz stress and prepare you for a perfect night's kip.
Cost: From £109
Find out more qhotels.co.uk/our-locations/the-midland-manchester/the-spa-at-the-midland

→

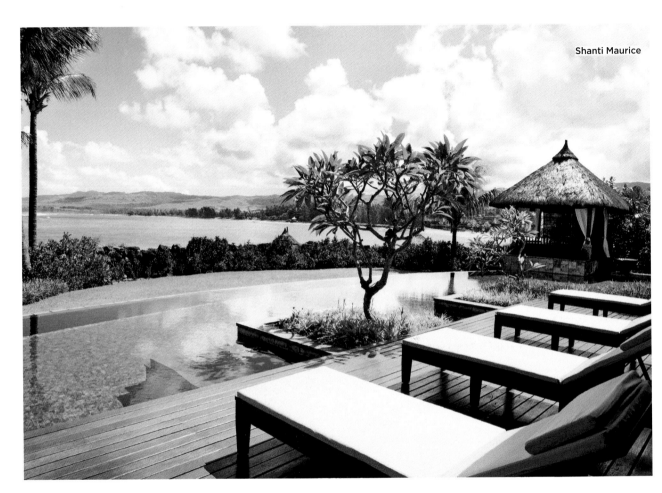

Shanti Maurice

Indulgent sleepy holidays

Have a bit of cash to splash and want to go abroad for your insomnia cure? Enjoy these gorgeous spas...

● **SHANTI MAURICE, MAURITIUS**
The stunning setting of this boutique Indian Ocean resort will immediately help you start to unwind. The spa's ayurvedic-inspired Shanti Sleep package comprises über-soothing yoga nidra with gentle stretching exercises and breathwork to lull your brain into a sleepy state. You'll also benefit from a range of gorgeous therapies including reflexology, magnesium sleep therapy and Tibetan sound massage. Ideal for blitzing stress if you've been through a difficult time, as well as for arming you with the tools you need to sleep well when you get home.
Cost: From £2,750 for five nights half-board, single person in a junior suite.
Find out more: shantimaurice.com

In ayurveda, your sleep disturbance relates to your dosha, or constitution. The busy mind of vata types stops them falling asleep. Pitta types drop off easily but wake in the night. A kapha will sleep, but wake feeling dull and lethargic

● **SHA WELLNESS CLINIC, SPAIN**

Okay, it isn't cheap, but if you're struggling with a serious long-term sleep problem, this award-winning wellness spa in beautiful Alicante may give you some answers. The bespoke Sleep Recovery Programme uses advanced medical techniques to record sleep quality and advise on ways to tackle problems. But for relaxation and pampering, you'll also get the best of Eastern knowledge with private yoga and mindfulness classes, dietary advice, massages and acupuncture. The programme can be tailored to deal with issues from insomnia to sleep apnoea.

Cost: From €3,500 for seven nights, including meals, consultations and treatments – but not accommodation. Mountain view deluxe suites start from €360 per night.

Find out more: shawellnessclinic.com

● **LEFAY RESORT & SPA, ITALY**

Set on gorgeous Lake Garda, this secluded sanctuary's Sleep Well programme is rooted in Chinese medicine and the idea that disrupted energy flow is what affects your sleep. So the five-night break is aimed at rebalancing it. First up, you'll have a consultation and personalised hormonal profiling to find out how your endocrine system affects your sleep patterns, and vice versa. Then it's onto the snooze-inducing therapies that will smooth out those energy pathways – acupuncture, reflexology, phytotherapies, heat therapies, outdoor tai chi and refreshing salt water lake therapy will leave you feeling relaxed by night and revitalised by day.

Cost: From £2,155 per person in a shared room for five nights, including all meals, return flights and transfers.

Find out more: healthandfitnesstravel.com/destinations/europe/italy/lefay/lefay-sleep-well

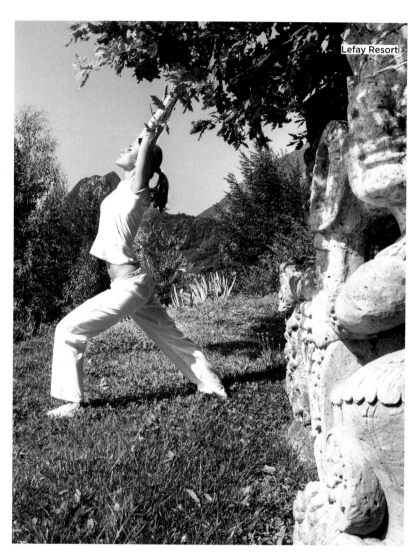
Lefay Resort

● **KAMALAYA WELLNESS SANCTUARY, THAILAND**

Choose from five, seven or nine nights to restore your long-term sleep pattern on the Sleep Enhancement programme at this blissful Koh Samui spa. Drawing on naturopathy, ayurveda and Chinese medicine, you'll enjoy treatments including shirodhara, an ayurvedic therapy involving the pouring of warm oil onto your forehead to deeply calm you. You'll also have massage, foot massage and acupuncture to help you relax.

Cost: From £3,320 per person for seven nights, including accommodation, flights and local transfers.

Find out more: thehealthyholidaycompany.co.uk/kamalaya-sleep-enhancement

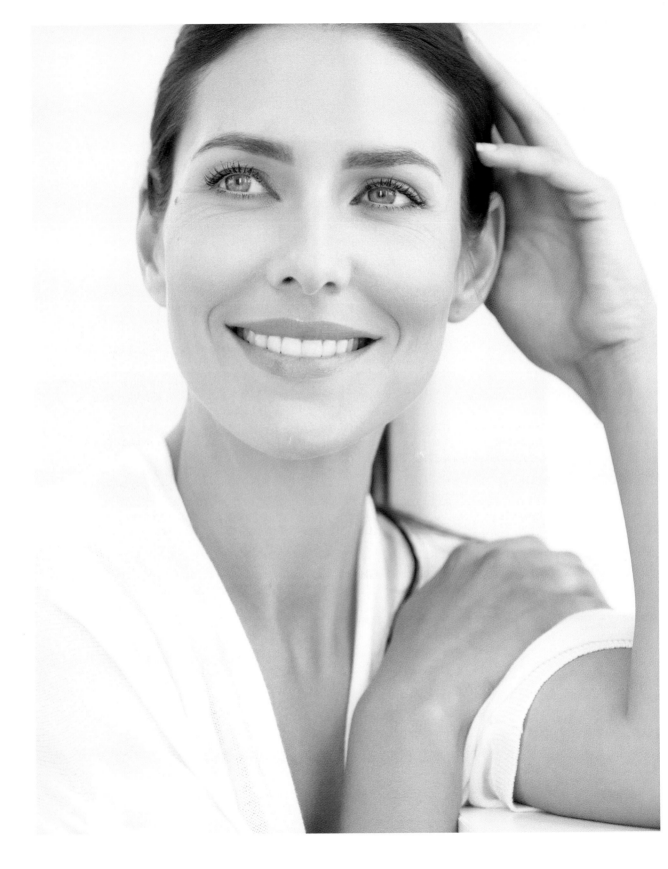

Directory

ADVICE

British Society of Clinical Hypnosis
bsch.org.uk

Everyone Active
everyoneactive.com

Open Focus Training
openfocusattentiontraining.com

The Sleep School
thesleepschool.org

The Sleep Council
sleepcouncil.org.uk

The British Wheel of Yoga
bwy.org.uk

Yogaia
yogaia.com

SUPPLEMENTS

A .Vogel
avogel.co.uk

Bach Rescue Night
nelsonsnaturalword.com

BetterYou
betteryou.com

CherryActive
cherryactive.co.uk

Higher Nature
highernature.co.uk

Nature's Best
naturesbest.co.uk

Pukka Herbs
pukkaherbs.com

Solgar
solgar.co.uk

Viridian
viridian-nutrition.com

PRODUCTS

Headspace
headspace.com

Lumie
lumie.com

Miaroma Relaxing Lavender Sleep Mist
hollandandbarrett.com

Silentnight
silentnight.co.uk

SlumberSlumber
slumberslumber.com

Tazeka aromatherapy
naturismo.com

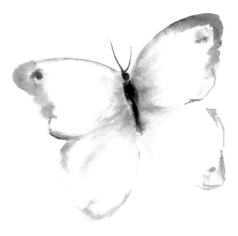

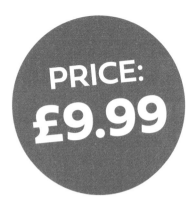
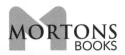

Kitchen Garden

Subscribe from £29*

Kitchen Garden is Britain's best guide to growing your own.

It offers down-to-earth advice from the finest minds in gardening to make sure you get the tastiest produce from your plot. There are tips on how to grow a wide range of fruit and vegetable crops and how to control troublesome pests plus what to do on your plot each month. Also buying guides, recipes and inspirational garden visits. Gardeners up and down the country share their experiences of sowing, growing and harvesting and every month KG has prizes and offers that could save you a fortune on a range of gardening essentials.

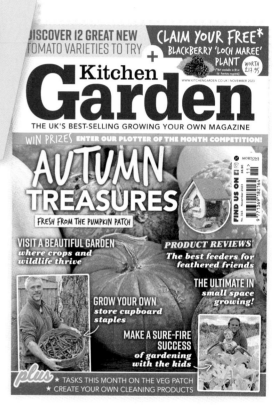

DISCOVER 12 GREAT NEW TOMATO VARIETIES TO TRY

CLAIM YOUR FREE* BLACKBERRY 'LOCH MAREE' PLANT WORTH £17.95

Kitchen Garden
THE UK'S BEST-SELLING GROWING YOUR OWN MAGAZINE

WIN PRIZES ENTER OUR PLOTTER OF THE MONTH COMPETITION!

AUTUMN TREASURES
FRESH FROM THE PUMPKIN PATCH

VISIT A BEAUTIFUL GARDEN where crops and wildlife thrive

PRODUCT REVIEWS The best feeders for feathered friends

THE ULTIMATE IN small space growing!

GROW YOUR OWN store cupboard staples

MAKE A SURE-FIRE SUCCESS of gardening with the kids

plus ★ TASKS THIS MONTH ON THE VEG PATCH ★ CREATE YOUR OWN CLEANING PRODUCTS

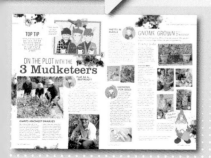

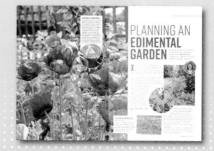

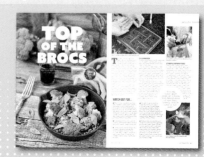

Sleep in numbers

7 THE NUMBER OF YEARS YOU SHOULD KEEP YOUR MATTRESS BEFORE REPLACING IT WITH A NEW ONE.

4pm should be the time you have your last caffeinated drink if you don't want it to affect your sleep that night, according to a study from Henry Ford Hospital and Wayne State College of Medicine in Detroit.

1 hr THE AMOUNT OF EXTRA SLEEP WOMEN NEED COMPARED TO MEN, RESEARCH HAS FOUND. SOME EXPERTS BELIEVE NOT GETTING IT IS ONE OF THE REASONS WOMEN MAY BE MORE LIKELY TO EXPERIENCE DEPRESSION.

1-in-3 of us experience sleepwalking at some point, according to one study from Stanford University School of Medicine in the US – far more than was once thought. Sleepwalking is associated with depression and excess alcohol intake, while those taking SSRI antidepressants were found to be three times more likely to sleepwalk in any one month.

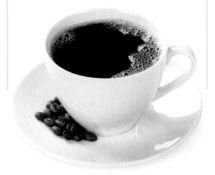

50% of your dream recollection goes within five minutes of waking – which is why, if you want to remember your brain's nocturnal wanderings, you should keep a dream diary beside your bed (see In your dreams, p 88).

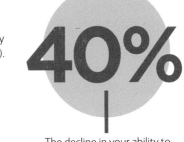

40% The decline in your ability to remember new things if you've had a bad night's sleep.

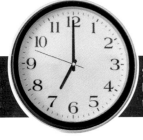

Six hours' sleep leads to double the amount of stress hormone cortisol circulating in your system, compared to sleeping for eight hours, German research found.